B. Jain's B.H.M.S.
SOLVED PAPERS
On
REPERTORY

DR. RITU ARORA
B.H.M.S. (Gold Medalist)
N.H.M.C. New Delhi

B. JAIN PUBLISHERS (P) LTD.
An ISO 9001 : 2000 Certified Company
USA — EUROPE — INDIA

B. JAIN'S B.H.M.S. SOLVED PAPERS ON REPERTORY

First Edition: 1993
10th Impression: 2010

> **Note from the Publishers**
> Any information given in this book is not intended to be taken as a replacement for medical advice. Any person with a condition requiring medical attention should consult a qualified practitioner or therapist.

All rights reserved. No part of this book may be reproduced, stored in a retrieval system or transmitted, in any form or by any means, mechanical, photocopying, recording or otherwise, without any prior written permission of the publisher.

© with the publisher

Published by Kuldeep Jain for
B. JAIN PUBLISHERS (P) LTD.
An ISO 9001 : 2000 Certified Company
1921/10, Chuna Mandi, Paharganj, New Delhi 110 055 (INDIA)
Tel.: +91-11-4567 1000 • *Fax:* +91-11-4567 1010
Email: info@bjain.com • *Website:* www.bjain.com

Printed in India

ISBN: 978-81-319-0521-0

DEDICATED TO MY PARENTS
AND MY FAMILY

CONTENTS

Sl. No.	Name of Chapter	Page No.
	Foreword	3
	Preface	4
1.	History of Repertory	5
2.	Case-Taking	13
3.	Symptoms	29
4.	Evaluation of Symptoms	45
5.	Choice of Repertory	55
6.	Steps of Repertorisation	61
7.	Kent's Repertory	67
8.	Boger's Characteristic Repertory	81
9.	Card Repertories	107
10.	Repertory in general	117
11.	Computers in Repertorisation	129

FOREWORD

The word ACCESS means APPROACH, THE WAY. This work of mine is a simple and easy way to study the repertory. This is meant specially for the students of both B.H.M.S. and D.H.M.S. who study this subject as a part of their academic curriculum.

"Oh! repertory! what a boring subject and moreover no material is available on this subject". These are the usual exclamations and problems of students studying repertory. This work is small but comprehensive and will prove very useful and beneficial for everybody with complete and uptodate information regarding the whole subject including use of computers in repertory. The presentation itself is unique. To understand the subject more deeply details have been discussed before starting the questions. I have tried with best of my efforts, knowledge and hard work to make it a valuable work.

Repertory is a difficult subject to understand and use but with repeated study the subject can be made easy to master.

I hope and wish that this work will be accepted and appreciated. Readers are welcome to make suggestions and point out errors or omissions if any to improve the work.

RITU ARORA

PREFACE

Repertory is a very neglected subject. Good literature on this subject is very scarce. I have put in all my sincere efforts to make this small book enlight the subject of repertory.

In this small work I have tried my level best to cover the whole subject with special emphasis on few aspects. The subject matter is updated and includes all possible information for the students ranging from curious to average who either want to achieve good marks in repertory or just to get through the examination.

For the complete mastery of the subject it is essential to go through the available repertories with an understanding of their basic principle. I have got the inspiration from my parents who encouraged me to bring out this work. (Preface)

In the end, I should not forget to thank Dr P.N. Jain and Mr Kuldeep Jain of M/s B. Jain Publishers for giving me an opportunity of writing this book. (Preface)

New Delhi   **RITU ARORA**

23-6-93

CHAPTER-I

HISTORY OF REPERTORY

The origin of repertory is as old as history itself. It owes itself to the dedicated efforts of the homoeopaths who were keenly interested in the upliftment of the science.

The origin of the repertory came with the index of **Fragmenta de Viribus Medicamentorum Positivis written in 1805.** Then a short clinical repertory came in 1817 compiled by Dr. Hahnemann which was not uptodate.

Today repertory has almost become an indispensable aid to the homoeopathic practitioners. The advent of repertory has facilitated the concentration and maximum utilization of the facts recorded in the numerous pages of homoeopathic literature.

In practical application, these numerous facts remained almost inaccessible or infrequently utilized for want of a suitable incorporation. Now many repertories have flooded the markets with different aims and approaches which has resulted in a large-scale progress in repertorisation.

Q-1. Give a brief history of repertories. (1990, 1992)

A-1. Today repertory has become almost an indispensable aid to the homoeopathic practitioners. A repertory is good only when its construction, arrangement and the author's directions for use are understood. We cannot understand the repertory unless we study the history and development of the repertory.

In addition, several mechanical methods are employed to make the repertory more approachable. A large variety of repertories based on different approaches and principles are available. It is quite interesting to know the origin and progress of the repertory.

CONCEPT OF REPERTORISATION: With Cinchona bark experiment Dr. Hahnemann introduced a new method of studying the qualities of a drug. With this commenced a new era in the field of pharmacy, with this was discovered the **'Law of Similars'**. He found that all the drugs which were known as specifics for certain diseases according to the orthodox medical system produced those very symptoms for which they were curative.

But the action of those drugs were recorded in the pharmacology in a very general way and in an incomplete form so that it was difficult to differentiate between the actions of the drugs belonging to the same group. So he decided to prove drugs on himself and others to get a fuller account of the positive effects of drugs on healthy human organisms.

This resulted in the production of 2 volumes of **Materia Medica Pura** and 5 volumes of **Chronic Diseases.** There was a gradual increase in the wealth of proved symptoms. The polychrest drugs' proved symptoms were not only difficult but impossible for a human mind to keep in store.

Then Dr. Hahnemann thought of compiling the symptoms in a broad-based work called **Repertory.**

The earlier repertory was born as early as 1805 when Hahnemann published in Latin his famous **'Fragmenta de Viribus Medicamentorum Positivis'**. The first part contained symptoms observed, and the second part formed the index or repertory.

STUDY OF REPERTORY

Dr. Hahnemann prepared the repertory after facing critical problems and wanted to get it published in 1830 but could not, as his publisher Mr. Arnold was not in a position to do so. It was called Hahnemann's referral material which had 4239 pages with four volumes in total. The pages had slits to hold little square papers of which he had cut out the corners so as to slip them into the slits and be able to change them in need.

In about 1829, he assigned a young doctor Ernst Ferdinand Ruckert to arrange a repertory of the remedies. This was to form the last volume of the Chronic Diseases. He worked on it from 1822 to 1830, his work being constantly checked and rechecked by Hahnemann, but the attempt could not be converted into a success. It remained in the manuscript form, placed now in the Haehl's Museum, Germany.

Till this time the idea of the repertory was very much confined and fixed in the mind of Dr. Hahnemann. So he employed Dr. Jahr in 1834 to complete the work again in a systematic and methodical way. Jahr was a medical student who had finished his medical course but had not appeared in the final examinations.

Dr. Hahnemann had set high hopes on him. But soon he began to complain of Jahr's hastiness and inexactitude. Jahr did not publish his repertory till 1835. His repertory was in German, with two volumes having 1052 and 1254 pages respectively. He had prepared a small repertory on bones, glands and mucous membranes consisting of 200 pages. His work was based on the alphabetical study of symptoms from the Chronic Diseases.

Although Hahnemann used his work for reference, but he did not stop here, and asked another student of his, Boenninghausen, to compile a complete work of repertory. He published the **"Repertory of Antipsorics"** in 1832, another **"Repertory of medicines that are not antipsoric"** in 1835. In 1836 he published **"Attempt at Showing the Relative Kinship of Homoeopathic Medicines"**. At last after a clinical experience of ten years he published a "**Therapeutic Manual**" in 1846, which had all the relevant information from his work and experience.

Actually the credit for giving birth to the repertory goes to Dr. Hahnemann although Jahr was the first person to get it published followed by Boenninghausen. In this way the progress of the repertory began.

Early references: Although many authors made serious attempts but could not succeed either because of lack of funds or due appreciation of their work.

Hahnemann's pupil Dr. Gross compiled two volumes of repertory which never appeared in the print. Later the work was taken over by Jahr, Ruckert and others without much success.

Finally a serious attempt was made by Boenninghausen. Boenninghausen's work can truly be considered as the beginning of new era in recognising repertory as an additional and indispensably valuable tool. His work kindled a new interest in the area of compiling repertories.

IMPORTANT YEARS IN THE HISTORY OF REPERTORY:

1832: Boenninghausen's Repertory of Antipsorics with a preface by Hahnemann.

1833: Glazer - First alphabetical repertory with 165 pages.

1835: Boenninghausen's Repertory of Medicines which are not Antipsoric.

1836: Boenninghausen's attempt to show the relative kinship of homoeopathic medicines. (Verwandschaften Repertorium)

STUDY OF REPERTORY

1837: Ruoff: A Repertory published at Stuttgart.

1843: Laffitte: A Homoeopathic Repertory of Symptomatology.

1845: Ruoff: A Repertory of Nosology.

Boenninghausen's Therapeutic Pocket Book.

1847: Hempel: Boenninghausen's Repertory.

1848: Clofar Muller: Systematic Alphabetical Repertory.

1849: Mure's Repertory.

1851: Bryant: An Alphabetical Repertory.

1853: Possart: A Repertory of Characteristic Homoeopathic Remedies.

1854: A. Lippe: Repertory of Comparative Materia Medica.

1859: Cipher Repertory by English homoeopaths.

Buck's Regional Repertory.

Hempel's Repertory.

Curie Repertory.

Hahnemann Society Repertory by Drysdale - Dudgeon.

1873: Berridge: Repertory of Eyes.

1874: Granier of Nimes: Homoeolexicon.

1879: C. Lippe: Repertory of the more characteristic symptoms.

1880: T.F. Allen: Symptom Register.

1881: Hering: Analytical Repertory.

1890: Gentry's Repertory of Concordances in six volumes.

1896: Knerr: The Repertory to Hering's Guiding Symptoms.

Era of Kent's repertory: During the last quarter of the 19th century the field of repertory became wider with unusually large number of repertories. The need of a new systematic repertory was felt. It led to the advent of Kent's Repertory in 1897. It was based entirely on different principle. It has been accepted as the most valuable document in the field of repertory.

Regional repertories: With the introduction of Kent's repertory the confusion was less, but the physicians needed a new change which could give them a short cut to prescribing. It was mainly because of the rapid evolution in the field of homoeopathy and the advancement of pathology and diagnosis. This led to the emergence of regional repertories shown below.

1873: Repertory of Eyes by Berridge.

Desires and Aversions by Guernsey.

1880: Repertory of Modalities by Worcester.

Repertory of Haemorrhoids by Guernsey.

Respiratory Organs by Lutze.

Repertory of Neuralgia by Lutze.

Repertory of Intermittent Fevers by W.A. Allen.

Repertory of Fevers by H.C. allen.

Repertory of Foot Sweat by O.M. Drake.

Repertory of sensations by Holcombe.

1884: Repertory of cough and expectoration by Lee and Clarke.

1892: Repertory of Digestive System by Arkell McMichell.

1894: Rep. of Rheumatism by Perkins.

Rep. of Therapeutics of Respiratory system by Vandenburg.

STUDY OF REPERTORY

      Rep. of Rheumatism by Pulford.

      Eczema by C.F. Mills Paugh.

      Headaches by Knerr.

      Appendicitis by Yingling.

      Repertory of Headaches by Neatby.

      Repertory of Labour by Yingling.

1906: Uterine Therapeutics by Minton.

      Repertory of Head by Nierhard.

      Shedd's Clinical Repertory,

      Bell's Diarrhoea.

      Boger's Time of Remedies.

      Repertory of urinary organs by A.R. Morgan.

      Repertory by P.F. Curie.

      Raue's Pathology.

      Boericke's Repertory.

      Repertory by Sarkar.

      Nash's Repertory of Respiratory Diseases.

      Clarke's Clinical Repertory.

      Repertory of Mastitis by Guernsey.

      Repertory of Throat by Guernsey.

Post-Kentian repertories: After the publication of Kent's *magnum opus*, very few repertories were published.

1904	-	Clarke's Clinical Repertory.
1928	-	Boger's Card Repertory.
1931	-	Repertory with Synoptic Key.
1937	-	Sensations as if by Roberts.
1959	-	Jugal Kishore's Card Repertory.
1982	-	Barthel and Will Klunker's Synthetic Repertory.

Dr. Patel's Autovisual Homoeopathic Repertory.

Gradually the "computer" repertories were introduced. In this way the repertory has travelled a lot with a hope that new and more efficient repertories will be introduced.

CHAPTER-2

CASE-TAKING

According to Dr. Dhawle "Case-taking is essentially a social intercourse between a physician and a patient under certain predetermined conditions".

Collection of data is the primary object of taking a case. Successful case-taking supplies the physician with all the evidence that is necessary to arrive at the proper verdict in respect of the trinity of Diagnosis, Prognosis and Treatment.

During the course of a successful clinical interview a happy relationship develops between the two. It has been technically termed as rapport. Establishment of rapport enables the physician to understand the patient as a personality, the problems that face him and above all, the solution that he has effected.

The free communication effects a release of inner tensions in the patient which has a considerable therapeutic value. Collection of data in the homoeopathic practice has thus developed into a higher, specialised technique calling for considerable skill on the part of the physician.

Q-1. What are the difficulties encountered usually in taking a chronic case? (1987. 1989 supp, 1990)

A-1. Case-taking is essentially a communication between the patient and the doctor. It provides all the possible information about the patient. The selection of the homoeopathic medicine depends on a good and elaborative case-taking. It is one of the tests for the success of a physician.

But many difficulties can be faced which can be either due to disease, patient or at times due to physician himself.

Let us discuss them one by one.

1. **DUE TO THE PATIENT:** It is one of the most prevailing significant factor which often comes as an obstacle for the physician. It is due to the many misunderstandings about the system of homoeopathy. But with the changing trends, this view has somewhat changed.

   a. **Nature of the patient:** The case-taking depends entirely on the free communication between the doctor and the patient, which is not possible in case of specially old people, infants, mentally retarded, unconscious patients and those who are unintelligent and non-cooperative.

   b. **Modesty hides the facts:** Although people are modernising and moving towards westernisation but still the patient feels shy to narrate some complaints to the doctor. This is seen specially when the doctor and the patient are of opposite sex and the matter relates to sex.

   It is seen in cases of sexually transmitted diseases, impotence, habitual masturbation, complaints related to coition, etc. Although patient may not think them to be of great significance but they definitely render a case-taking incomplete.

   c. **Pretension by the patient:** Pretention usually signifies a form of modification. It reflects the inner nature of the patient. Some patients are too timid and bashful and hide their symptoms or give them wrongly. But some are of different type, usually hysterical personalities who exaggerate their symptoms to gain the sympathy of the doctor. Both categories of the patients form a hindrance.

   d. **Long sufferings considered incurable:** We know that a chronic case usually requires an elaborative case-taking.

During the progress phase of the disease, many new symptoms appear, old ones disappear, with the intake of multiple number of medicines, which is considered as a new disease by the patient. Therefore he takes the treatment for the new ones, ignoring or considering as incurable the old ones. They are not usually revealed before the doctor thus giving only a one sided case presentation.

e. **Habituated to long sufferings:** In a chronic disease, the patients usually narrate the recently appeared changes in body and mind, but forget to explain or give any importance to the old symptoms to which they get accustomed. Since it is a feeling that long lasting symptoms may remain for life, they are not narrated, hence giving an obstacle to cure.

f. **Periodically appearing symptoms not narrated:** There are few patients who suffer from some symptoms which appear with a strong periodicity, such as complaints occurring in a particular season only, like spring, autumn, etc., or appearing after a fixed time interval. Such symptoms are ignored by the patient thus depriving the physician from the selection of a proper medicine.

g. **Alternating symptoms not narrated:** There are few patients who have alternation of one symptom with the other, out of which usually one is more troublesome than the other.

The patient usually does not understand that the two symptoms are the phases of one disease which are alternating with each other. Therefore, considering them as separate entities, he takes treatment for them separately, thereby obliterating this significant symptom.

h. **Self-medication:** It has now become a trend to take self-treatment. If the patient gets well, then he does not knock at the door of the doctor. But if the symptoms remain, he peeps into the clinic. As a result of prolonged self-medication the symptoms remain suppressed and pose a problem for the physician.

2. **DUE TO THE PHYSICIAN:** As we have seen above that a patient can create obstacles in a case-taking, similarly a physician can also create hindrances.

a. **Nature of physician:** If a physician is prejudiced, non-observant, careless and not dedicated or he himself does not feel confident then he cannot take the case properly. If he does not follow the norms of case-taking he can complicate the case.

b. **Unhomoeopathic medicines:** There are few categories of prescribers who give combined medicines, compounds, complexes, mixtures and external ointments which in a long run produce their own symptomatology thereby giving an entirely different picture of the disease, which for another physician becomes difficult to sort out.

3. **DUE TO THE DISEASE:**

a. **Suppression of disease:** There are many ways of treating a patient but only a single method to cure. In the different modes multiple medicines, complexes and ointments are given which cause the suppression of the disease, with appearance of new symptoms and disappearance of old ones thereby obscuring the true nature of the disease.

b. **Due to advanced pathology of the disease:** As we know that the prescription depends on a well framed case. But with the advancement of disease pathology develops and progresses, the basic symptomatology diminishes with the appearance of pathologic symptomatology.

c. **Complex diseases:** They are usually representative of a meagre symptomatology thereby causing difficulty in proper case-taking.

d. **Mixed miasmatic diseases:** There are few chronic diseases which have a combination of the miasms psora, sycosis and syphilis in a complex, vitiated form which is difficult to penetrate.

e. **One sided diseases:** They are a type of disease which presents too few symptoms for a judicious prescription.

Dr. Hahnemann has very clearly mentioned regarding the obstacles in Section 82-90 of the 5th edition of "Organon of Medicine".

Q-2. What is the importance of accurate record keeping in homoeopathic practice.? (1988 suppl.)

A-2. Record: It is essentially a written document of great significance depicting the patient as a whole and his symptomatology along with the treatment given.

One finds many medical practitioners who do not care to maintain any records except the prescription and the charges. Some maintain a semblance of record by noting down a few complaints.

A systematic clinical record is quite a rarity in private medical practice. One cannot rely on one's memory to that extent.

Homoeopathic practice demands all attention to the details that enable individualisation, but it rarely happens. Dr. Hahnemann states that a true homoeopathic physician is recognised by his characteristic method of enquiry in which he goes into the minutest details and puts them down carefully.

A well maintained clinical record leads to the development of a sound clinical acumen, furnishes the best possible material for clinical teaching, research, etc. and provides a reliable evidence of one's integrity and efficiency.

ADVANTAGES AND USEFULNESS OF RECORD KEEPING:

1. **PROPER ASSESSMENT OF THE CASE:** It plays a very significant role specially in chronic diseases where there

is a complex, vitiated picture. Without it a physician is not able to assess whether the patient has predominance of syphilitic, sycotic or psoric background.

Therefore a proper record helps in the assessment of the disease.

2. **SELECTION OF SECOND PRESCRIPTION:** after the first visit when the patient next comes to the physician the prescription has to be repeated, changed or potency to be altered, depending on the case. For this purpose the case record has to be referred to.

3. **FOLLOW UP OF CASES:** In chronic diseases, the patient has to take the treatment for a long period, which involves constant follow up of the case. Therefore case record is helpful.

4. **JUDGEMENT OF THE ACTION OF REMEDY:** When the patient is given some medicine, some change in the symptomatology is expected, e.g., new symptoms appear, old symptoms reappear, disappearance of new symptoms, etc. They all indicate the action of the medicine. This can be better analysed if we have an accurate clinical record.

5. **FOR PROVING THE SUPERIORITY OF THE SYSTEM:** There are different systems of medicine in the field of diseases, with a run of competition everywhere. Therefore if a physician cures some incurable or a rare, strange disease then the case record can be a documentary piece of evidence to prove the superiority of the system rather than making false claims.

6. **AS A REFERENCE:** Some patients are not regular in their treatment or some patients get cured of one disease and come back to the physician for some other disease after a long time. In any of the circumstances if the case record is maintained properly then it can help the physician to tackle the new problem smoothly.

7. IN LEGAL PROCEDURES: There are few patients who make false complaints against the attending physician. In such cases the doctor may be sued legally. Here comes the protection by a well maintained record, as a documentary evidence in favour of the physician.

8. ADDITION OF FRESH SYMPTOMS: As the patient comes regularly to the clinic, he always gives some new symptoms, or a change in the previous symptoms which can be added if the doctor has maintained a record.

9. FINDINGS OF EXAMINATION AND LAB INVESTIGATIONS: Clinical diagnosis is advancing with the introduction of new techniques for examination of the patient and laboratory investigations. These findings can be accommodated from time to time if a case record has been maintained.

10. FOR CLINICAL TEACHINGS: A well maintained case record can efficiently serve in the clinical teachings if some good cases have been elicited and recorded properly in details with follow-ups, mode and line of treatment along with any change in symptomatology.

11. REFLECTS THE SKILL OF THE PHYSICIAN: It is a reliable evidence of the integrity and efficiency of the doctor, his quality of thoroughness and dedication.

12. FOR RESEARCH PURPOSES: If it is a well preserved document with all possible details it is very useful for research and further progress of the system.

13. MISCELLANEOUS: Although a clinical record l multiple purposes but above all we say that it helps in arriving at a similimum after making complete analysis and synthesis of the case, thus fulfilling the mission of a good physician.

Q-3. A proper case-taking is a must for correct repertorisation. Discuss. (1985)

A-3. As we know collection of data pertaining to totality of symptoms is the most significant purpose of case-taking. For the right homoeopathic prescription a case has to be taken in all its details.

Therefore a complete case-taking is very essential as it serves multiple purposes of the physician.

1. **FRAMING THE TOTALITY OF SYMPTOMS:** A case if complete in all respects helps in the framing of a case totality which helps the physician in selection of medicine.

2. **TO PERCEIVE THE TRUE PICTURE:** A well taken case is a true picture of the disease, whether the symptoms are real or exaggerated to gain the attention of the physician.

3. **KNOWLEDGE OF DISEASE:** The disease manifests itself through signs and symptoms. If a case is taken then the symptoms can be separated as those of the patient and of the disease, thereby enhancing the knowledge of disease and of medicine.

4. **TO FIND OUT THE NATURE OF DISEASE:** Homoeopathy plays an important role both in acute and chronic diseases. But the nature and presentation of both differ from each other. Therefore it helps in the differentiation, treatment and prognosis of the case

5. **MODE OF DEVELOPMENT OF DISEASE:** Homoeopathic case-taking deals with the disease from its earliest available stage. It helps in knowing the mode of appearance of symptoms, their chronological sequence with any observed changes in them.

6. **CAUSATION OF DISEASE:** Homoeopathy offers different modes of prescribing. One of the ways is to prescribe on the basis of aetiology; exciting, maintaining or precipitating cause of the disease. So if a case is taken in details, then the cause can be elicited and utilised for prescription.

7. ANALYSIS AND EVALUATION OF SYMPTOMS:

This is the most significant purpose of case-taking.

Usually when a case is taken the symptoms are divided into the respective groups of common, uncommon, physical or mental symptoms.

With the completion of analysis, the symptoms are valuated according to their intensity and importance in the respective grades.

In fact all these points are essential for a complete case-taking leading to correct repertorisation.

Q-4. Describe the method of taking a chronic case and the difficulties involved in it. (1984)

A-4. The case-taking for a chronic case can be described under the following headings:

1. **PRE-REQUISITES:** These are some of the conditions which a physician should keep in mind.

    a. Proper sitting arrangement. Comfortable and adequate sitting accommodation.

    b. In the waiting room, suitable reading material should be provided.

    c. Adequate arrangement for light.

    d. Quietness and privacy are essential.

    e. Good mental attributes of the physician.

2. **OBSERVATIONS TO BE MADE:**

    a. General appearance of the patient, physical and mental.

b. Mental attitude of the patient, whether sad, depressed, quarrelsome or anxious, etc.

c. How the patient speaks, whether in a low tone, hoarse voice or brassy voice.

d. Condition of the pupils whether dilated or contracted.

e. Any discharge from the body.

f. Sweating: with character, whether increased or diminished, with or without odour, whether staining the clothes?

g. Salivation.

h. Condition of hair, face and nails, whether hair tangled, face pale or lively, etc.

Anaemia, cyanosis, paronychia can be assessed by examining the nails.

i. Any weakness noticed from the way the patient enters the clinic, the way she gets up from the chair, the way she drops into the chair, etc.

j. Even the miasms in the background can be ascertained from the way the patient narrates her complaints.

3. **TECHNIQUE OF INTERROGATION:** The case has to be taken in the following sequential order:

a. **Particulars of the patient:** It includes the name, age, sex of the patient along with the occupation, residential address, religion and the marital status.

b. **Present complaints:** The most important requisite for this is to note down the complaints in the language of the patient.

Each symptom should be qualified by its location, sensation, modality and concomitants.

STUDY OF REPERTORY

The physical generals should be enquired into in details. They are discussed below:

1. **Time modality:** Morning, evening, afternoon, etc.

2. **Circumstantial modality:** Any anxiety, physical or mental trauma, etc.

3. **Seasonal modality:** Summer, autumn, winter, spring etc.

4. Relation with eating, whether before, during or after meals. Any particular food which makes him worse or gives relief.

5. **Sleep:** With special reference to dreams and the particular position of body in sleep.

6. Any known etiology whether physical or mental with any known precipitating factor.

c. **History of present illness:** It specially deals with the etiology behind the onset of disease. How the disease progressed along with the appearance of symptoms in a chronological order or the disappearance of any symptoms.

d. **Past history:** It plays a very important role in finding the miasmatic background of the patient.

In this special reference has to be given to the following points.

1. History of any prolonged illness in the past, like recurrent urinary tract infection, tonsillitis, mental trauma, tuberculosis, diabetes, asthma, S.T.D., recurrent malaria, typhoid, etc.

2. **Birth history:** It includes prematurity, postmaturity, birth trauma, asphyxia, cyanosis, jaundice, congenital defects, etc.

3. History of development milestones, whether normal or abnormal.

4. History of vaccination with or without any untoward reaction.

5. History of any surgical interference, exposure to X-rays, etc.

6. Special reference should be given to the domestic circumstances, negligence, attitude of the parents, overprotection, relationship between father and mother.

e. **Family history:** It usually helps in deciding the miasmatic background. For this any evidence of true miasmatic disease in the family including parents, grandparents, sisters, brothers, paternal and maternal relations should be thoroughly noted.

Any evidence of T.B., diabetes mellitus, diabetes insipidus, cancer, allergic rhinitis, bronchial asthma, eczema, rheumatoid arthritis, schizophrenia, suicidal tendencies should be recorded.

f. **Personal history :** It usually deals with the personal identity of the patient. In general it includes the habits of smoking, alcoholism, extramarital relations, etc.

But in males special reference should be made of the following.

1. History of extramarital relations.

2. Any incidence of masturbation, impotency, etc.

In females thorough interrogation should be done to elicit the obstetrical and gynaecological history.

1. **GYNAECOLOGICAL HISTORY**: It includes the menarche, the duration of cycles, their character, any abnormality in the menstrual cycle.

STUDY OF REPERTORY

Any history of leucorrhoea, post-coital complaints, etc.

2. **OBSTETRICAL HISTORY:** It includes

    a.   The number of conceptions.

    b.   Whether all the trimesters were normal.

    c.   Any liking for any strange things during pregnancy or any particular aversion.

    d.   Any history of jaundice, bleeding per vagina, urinary tract infection during pregnancy.

    e.   Whether all the deliveries were normal. If not, then forceps or caesarean.

    f.   Any history of puerperal infection.

    g.   Whether she breast fed all the babies for normal duration.

    g.   **Treatment history:** In homoeopathy, it matters a lot to know the previous treatment. Whether the patient had been kept on oral corticosteroids, topical applications, prolonged antibiotics, and any untoward effect known of these drugs.

    h.   **Physical examination:** In the end, although it is not a part of case-taking, but without this examination the case-taking is not complete. It includes the complete examination of all the systems under the respective headings of inspection, palpation, percussion and auscultation.

In the end, it can be summed up with the special precautions given by Dr. Hahnemann in the "Organon of Medicine".

Do's	**Dont's**
1. Ask for all the complaints in details.	1. Do not put leading questions or questions which suggest an answer to the patient.
2. Speak slowly and write methodically.	2. Do not throw the questions in a haphazard manner.
3. Each symptom should be started in a fresh line.	3. Do not use complex or technical language and medical terms.
4. Symptoms should be noted in chronological order.	4. Do not hide anything from the patient.
5. You should be unprejudiced in observation and have complete dedication.	5. Do not rely on the patient's statements entirely. Always confirm it by cross interrogation.

In this way case-taking is a detailed, methodic technique in homoeopathy which requires capability, intelligence and patience on the part of both the patient and the physician.

For second part See Q-1 of Chapter-2.

Q-5. What is Case Recording? Write about it's usefulness and importance. (1986)

A-5. See Q-2. of Chapter-2. P-12

Q-6. Write short notes on:

1. Recording of cases and usefulness of recording (1989)

   A-1. See Q-2, Chapter-2. P-12

2. Methods of Record Keeping (1983)

STUDY OF REPERTORY 27

A-2. When the patient has not submitted any written history, the physician is required to make notes either when the patient is narrating his story or subsequently.

There are many methods of writing and maintaining records. They are:

1. **SPECIMEN INDEX CARDS:** They are the simplest form of cards employed for recording. These cards of same size are numbered or arranged alphabetically.

CASE REF. NO.	SPACE FOR INDEX LETTER	
Name	Age	Sex
Occupation		
Address		
Diagnosis		
Remedy		
Result		

2. **BOUND REGISTER:** It is a common way of record keeping which does not require any clerical assistance. In this, cases are arranged datewise with folio number in the register.

It usually suits the private practitioners.

Disadvantage: Record of the chronic case is scattered as the case is transferred from one folio to another register.

3. **LOOSE-LEAF FOLDER OR CARD SYSTEM:** Now it is the most followed mode of maintaining the case

records. It gives record reference on a large scale, therefore useful in big institutions and hospitals.

ADVANTAGES:

1. Cases are arranged serially or alphabetically.

2. Record of a chronic case is available at one place.

3. Records of the members of one family can be located in a single folder.

4. It is a flexible system with the advantage that if the number of patients increase they can be accommodated easily.

DISADVANTAGES:

1. Initial cost is more.

2. It essentially requires clerical assistance.

CHAPTER-3

SYMPTOMS

Almost every case that comes to the attention of the physician presents two distinct parts. One, the symptoms which are most annoying to the patient and most outstanding in his recognition. Secondly, those symptoms which he does not recognise as symptoms or which he does not consider worth reporting or does not consider as having relationship to the case.

The word symptom has been derived from the Greek word **"Symptoma"** which means "anything that happens", meaning any change in the health which is felt by the patient himself, remarked by those around him and observed by the physician.

According to Dr. Hahnemann, "It is the outward reflection of the internal essence of the disease, which is the affection of vital force."

According to Dr. Kent, "Every symptom is indicative of a deviation from the normal state of health".

According to Dr. Stuart Close, "In general a symptom is any evidence of disease, or change from a state of health".

According to Dr. Wright, "Symptoms to the homoeopaths are the language of body expressing its disharmony and calling for the similar remedy".

Knowledge of the true nature and constituent of a symptom is necessary in proving or testing medicines, in the examination of a patient, in the study of materia medica and in the selection and management of the indicated remedy.

Dr. Hahnemann defines it as any manifestation of a deviation from a former state of health, perceptible by the patient, the individuals around him or the physician.

He further defines symptom as "evidences of the operation of the influences which disturb the harmonious play of functions, the vital principle as a **Spiritual Dynamis**".

They constitute the only direct avenue of approach to that inner sphere which must otherwise remain closed to our investigation, except as it is indirectly revealed in certain automatic or involuntary objective symptoms from which accurate deductions can be made.

Q-1. Define general symptoms. What is their value in comparison to the particular symptoms? Describe in brief all the general symptoms to be taken into consideration for the repertorisation (1987).

Ans-1. General symptoms: The symptoms which depict an individual or represent him as a whole are called the general symptoms. They are those that affect the patient as a whole showing the picture of his disease in the mental and physical planes. While referring to them, the patient tends to use the word "I" and not "my".

But under certain conditions a particular symptom can also behave as a general symptom.

Value of general symptoms: The general symptoms are of immense diagnostic value specially of the patient. As Dr. Kent has rightly said, "they depict the EGO of the individual, therefore, assume a strong value".

1. They relate to the highest esteem of self which represents the ego.

2. They help in framing a totality and also help in the individualisation.

3. If these are strange, rare and peculiar they help in the selection of the similimum.

Categorisation of general symptoms: These general symptoms can be studied under physical generals and mental generals.

MENTAL GENERALS: They depict the ego of the mind. The mind enjoys importance over the body. Therefore these symptoms are of highest value.

They can be categorised as:

1. Will and emotion.
2. Intellect and understanding.
3. Memory.

Will and emotion: They enjoy the highest position as they reflect the core of the mind. They usually manifest in the form of loves, hates, suicidal tendencies, fears, desire or aversion to company, suspicion, etc.

The components of will are

    a. **External will:** It is usually voluntary and responds to the external influences, tempting the person to do or not to do things.

    b. **Internal will:** It is the conscience which is the deepest of all and is unchanged by the medicines.

Emotions provide the greatest driving force to an individual. A proper understanding is very essential for a physician absorbed in a critical evaluation of an individual's total response to his surroundings.

The emotional state manifests itself in various ways.

1. Direct expression: Through appropriate feelings.

2. Indirect expression: through

   a. **Opposite feelings:** The original emotions evoke a strong feeling of guilt and this prevents direct expression.

   b. **Disturbed functioning:** through

   1. Voluntary nervous system.

   2. Autonomic nervous system.

   3. Endocrine system.

   c. **Dreams:** They reflect the unconscious drives and aspirations.

Intellect and understanding: It determines the individual capacity of the person while the emotions determine their free expression.

The emotions assume the pride of place when we try to assess an individual's susceptibility to illness and visualise the picture of the disease. The functions of the intellect can be considered under the following categories.

1. **Perception of environment:** In addition to sensory perception it includes the function of discrimination and interpretation.

2. Formulation of ideas, thoughts, concepts, etc.

3. **Discrimination:** The freedom of choice gives the ability to distinguish between the right and the wrong.

4. **Action:** Volition enables to pursue the right path. They can be summed up as:

a. Aberrations of perception and disturbances of formulation: hallucinations, delusions, illusions, confusion of ideas, etc.

b. **Disturbances of discrimination and volition:** Confusion, indecisiveness; destructive impulses such as homicidal, suicidal, etc.

Memory: This is a part of the intellect but is dealt with seperately. It manifests as the loss of memory either complete or partial, for the names of persons, places, etc.

Physical generals: They are the symptoms on the physical plane of the person as a whole. The common physical generals are discussed.

1. **Reaction to environment:** It usually shows the sensitivity of an individual to the environmental stimuli. The patient can be either very sensitive to cold, chilly or can be very sensitive to the heat or can be sensitive to both the extremes. Can be even insensitive to both extremes of temperature.

2. **Sensations and complaints in general:** These deal with the sensations experienced by the patient in the physical plane. It also enlists few objective conditions including coldness or hotness of hands, feet, etc.

3. **Relation with eating:** This includes any relation whether before, after or during the eating and any particular food element which causes disturbance in the entire system.

This also includes the desires and aversions which are highly helpful in distinguishing one patient from the other.

4. **Sleep:** Normally the rest that one obtains in sleep proves refreshing and a restful sleep is one which the patient looks

forward to. However, when one sees its reverse—the patient who wakes up all cross and irritable, the patient who wakes up in the morning none the better and still fagged out, the patient who wakes into an aggravation of all his complaints, it assumes a great importance as one of the characteristic features of the case. A very striking amelioration of the complaints after even a small nap is a rare symptom and hence a significant symptom.

Special importance should be given to the position during sleep, snoring and mumbling during sleep.

5. **Sexual instincts:** The sexual drive is one of the basic instincts which promotes the continuation of race. Any affection of it or any aggravation of troubles during or after sexual act will be of great importance.

Similarly in females special emphasis should be given to the menstruation—its duration, character and any notable aggravation or amelioration during the flow.

Any abnormality in the sexual impulse should be noted. In females due importance should be given to the ailments during pregnancy and puerperium.

6. **Symptoms relating to special senses:** These are the symptoms showing under the category of speech, hearing, vision, sense of smell, etc.

Although all the symptoms have been discussed but sometimes a particular symptom behaves as a general symptom. In such circumstances the independent decision and knowledge of the physician is to be reckoned.

7. **Pathological generals:** Boger emphasised these symptoms. They usually relate to general tendencies of the tissues and propensity to certain types of abnormal changes which feature in selecting the remedy. It includes:

EASE TO DISEASE

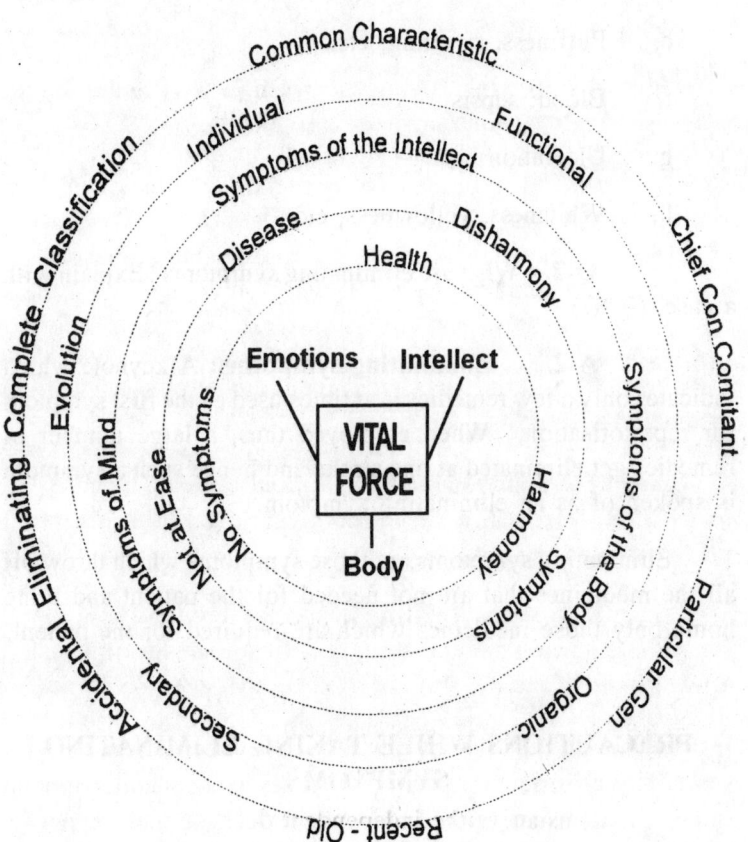

a. Calculi

b. Cysts

c. Fibrous tissue - fibroma

d. Haemorrhage

e. Puffiness, swelling, etc.

f. Blood: sepsis

g. Ulceration

h. Whiteness, yellowness, etc.

Q-2. What are eliminating symptoms? Explain with a case. (1987)

A-2. **Eliminating symptoms:** A keynote which indicates only a few remedies is at times used as the first symptom for repertorisation. When employed thus, a large number of remedies get eliminated at one stroke and hence such a symptom is spoken of as an eliminating symptom.

Eliminating symptoms are those symptoms which throw off all the medicines that are not needed for the patient and bring home only those medicines which are required for the patient.

PRECAUTIONS WHILE TAKING ELIMINATING SYMPTOMS

1. The symptom selected should be real and of marked intensity, expressing the inner need of the patient.

2. The symptoms should be arranged in their order of importance so that a peculiar, uncommon symptom can be selected.

STUDY OF REPERTORY

3. We must be sure that the symptom chosen should cover the whole man and not express him superficially.

How to proceed: First of all the symptom which is peculiar, uncommon and most expressive of all should be selected. This symptom is placed at the top and rest of the symptoms below it. The medicines that are not covered by the first symptom, that is, the one placed at the top, will be eliminated from the rest of the symptoms.

ADVANTAGE OF ELIMINATION:

It acts as a safe short cut to prescription in the hands of experienced physicians who have learnt to mind the generals.

An example: A male patient aged 32 years had developed suddenly pain in right big toe. Although he had pain but there was no swelling or any other local findings. All his investigations were done to rule out gout and the rheumatic diathesis.

The case was taken in detail, although nothing specifically came out regarding the onset of the problem. The pain was worse only when standing and mild walking but he used to feel better if he exerted like playing badminton or running very rapidly.

He was of neurotic type but with extreme anger and anxiety. He used to be very anxious for the anger bursts, while he lost his temper there was lot of trembling all over the body.

The most significant point was that as soon as the pain started he used to have **"dreams of urinating"**. Even when he used to have a nap the same phenomenon occurred.

He gave the explanation that his grandfather and father had diabetes, and that's why he was having these thoughts running in sleep. But even when their diabetes was under control, he used to dream the same way.

At the end his mother added that he was very fond of sweets but now the desire is gradually waning. He is otherwise a computer operator with sitting job and no tension. The case-taking concluded with the strange sensation of plug in throat during sleep.

The case was worked out in the following manner.

1. Desire for sweets
2. Dreams of urinating
3. Pain big toe better by physical exertion and rapid walking but worse on standing
4. Angered easily
5. Trembling during anger
6. Anxiety during anger
7. Sensation of plug in throat during sleep

From all these the dreams of urinating was taken as the eliminating symptom.

	SYMPTOMS	Ambr	Kreos	Lac can	Lyc	M.I.F.	Seneg	Sep	Sulph
1.	DREAMS OF URINATING	1	2	1	1	1	2	2	1
2.	DESIRES SWEETS	-	-	-	3	-	-	2	3
3.	SENSATION OF PLUG	-	-	-	-	-	-	2	-
4.	TREMBLING, ANGER, DURING	1	-	-	-	-	-	-	-
5.	ANXIETY, ANGER, DURING	-	-	-	-	-	-	1	-

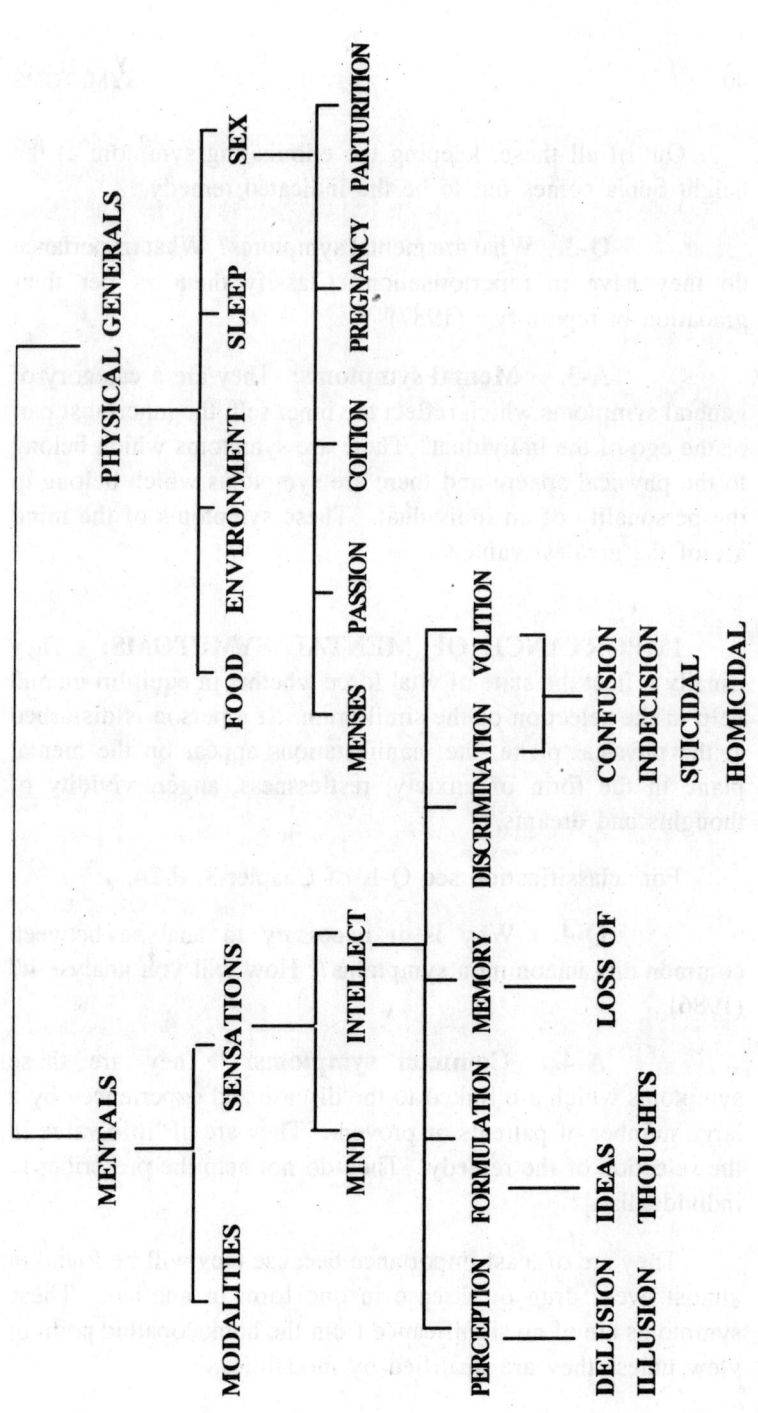

Out of all these, keeping the eliminating symptom at the height Sepia comes out to be the indicated remedy.

Q-3. What are mental symptoms? What importance do they have in repertorisation? Classify them as per their gradation in repertory. (1987)

A-3. Mental symptoms: They are a category of general symptoms which reflect the inner self, the innermost part or the ego of the individual. There are symptoms which belong to the physical sphere and there are symptoms which belong to the personality of an individual. These symptoms of the mind are of the greatest value.

IMPORTANCE OF MENTAL SYMPTOMS: They usually reflect the state of vital force whether in equilibrium and help in the selection of the similimum. If a person is disturbed at the physical plane, the manifestations appear on the mental plane in the form of anxiety, restlessness, anger, vividity of thoughts and dreams.

For classification see Q-1. of Chapter-3. P-24.

Q-4. Why is it necessary to analyse between common and uncommon symptoms? How will you analyse it? (1986)

A-4. Common symptoms: They are those symptoms which are linked to the disease and experienced by a large number of patients or provers. They are of little value in the selection of the remedy. They do not help the prescriber to individualise.

They are of least importance because they will be found in almost every drug or disease in one form or another. These symptoms are of no significance from the homoeopathic point of view unless they are qualified by modalities.

For example, aching soreness, nausea, vomiting loss of appetite, weakness, constipation, etc. But if they get modified by uncommon modalities they become important. For example, trembling or weakness before stool, constipation before and during menses, loss of appetite during menses, etc.

UNCOMMON SYMPTOMS: They are explained by the formula of P,Q,R,S, peculiar, queer, rare and strange. It denotes those symptoms which are:

1. Peculiar in their nature and character

2. Where no explanation is possible

3. Which are peculiar to a few patients suffering from similar diseases.

4. Their presence cannot be explained on the basis of pathology.

5. They have their basis in the constitutional make-up that determines the psyche of the individual.

6. They usually help in the miasmatic understanding of the case.

Why to analyse the two:

1. To individualise a case.

2. For the selection of the similimum.

3. For framing an altogether different totality to serve the purpose of repertorisation.

These symptoms can be analysed only if one has thorough knowledge of the symptomatology. If one has complete understanding of case-taking, evaluation and the synthesis of the case then they can be easily analysed and can be made as a turning point for the selection of similimum. This essentially requires the complete knowledge of the medicine, and of diseases, the expertise by which the symptoms belonging to the patient and those of the disease can be differentiated and analysed.

Q-5. Write short notes on:

    a.   Concomitant symptoms (1987, 1988, 1988 supp, 1990)

    b.   General and particular symptoms (1988 supp.)

    c.   Complete symptom (1988 supp, 1989 supp)

Ans-4.

A. **Concomitant symptoms:** The symptoms that accompany the chief complaints are called the concomitant symptom. The word concomitant means existing or occurring together. They are also known as **associated or auxiliary symptoms.**

The concomitants bear no other relationship to the chief complaint than this time association. When these symptoms cannot be explained by pathology they become characteristic symptoms.

They usually represent the individual reactions and therefore the prescription in homoeopathic practice. Concomitants arise from the inherent constitutional aspects and tend to remain constant with a patient irrespective of the nature of the disease.

Dr. Boenninghausen was the first to realise the importance of the concomitants in prescribing and constructing his repertory. Boger developed this idea fully in Boenninghausen's Characteristics and Repertory with additions and modifications.

B. **General symptoms:** See Q-1 of Chapter-3. P-24.

Particular symptoms: The symptoms which are related to a particular part, organ or function of the body are called particular or local symptoms. They are narrated by the patient with the prefix 'my', e.g., my head, my stomach, etc.

STUDY OF REPERTORY

These symptoms tend to disturb the patient most and he seeks consultation for them only. The general constitutional symptoms usually recede under the circumstances so that they are perceived, if at all, in a hazy manner. Thus the prescription of acute necessity will be based on these particulars. In rare instances this does not obtain and the general constitutional symptoms come to the forefront.

It should be appreciated that the generals help in the delineation of the outline whereas the particulars furnish the details to differentiate the remedies.

IMPORTANCE:

1. At times a peculiar, strong particular may point to a small group of remedies and thus help a quick prescription. In this way it acts as a keynote.

2. According to Boenninghausen they provide a base for the evolution of generals, hence their importance.

3. When a particular symptom is experienced at more than two places, it behaves as a general and becomes important.

C. **Complete symptom:** The incomplete symptom is one which lacks any of the four elements of location, sensation, modality and concomitants. This particular defect was noticed first by Boenninghausen. Therefore he advocated the concept of complete symptom. Symptom which is clearly defined by the elements of location, sensation, modality and concomitants is called a complete symptom.

This is further modified on the principles of analogy given by Dr. Boenninghausen.

1. **Location:** It points to the exact situation or localisation of the complaint.

2. **Sensation:** Any altered perception of the mind

regarding the disease. It is manifested either in the form of pains, aches or any discomfort felt both physically as well as mentally.

3. **Modality:** Anything which modifies a symptom for better or worse is called the modality. It can be in terms of time, place, climate, or any circumstances.

4. **Concomitants:** The symptom associated with the chief complaint is called a concomitant. For example, while coughing spurting of urine, while urinating increased salivation.

CHAPTER-4

EVALUATION OF SYMPTOMS

After painstaking enquiry the physician has accumulated a mass of data which threatens to engulf him. He has to classify and grade them in order to give it a form.

This form will have to depict truly the patient as a whole which at the same time will readily reveal its counterpart in the materia medica.

Evaluation of symptoms means the principle of grading or ranking of different symptoms in order of value which are to be matched with the drug symptoms in order to superimpose a similar drug disease on the characteristic totality of the natural disease.

As a result of years of clinical experience pooled together, a system of evaluation has been evolved which finds ready acceptance in the field of repertorisation.

Proper evaluation of symptoms is the most important step next to case-taking in homoeopathy. In analysis of a case, the value of symptoms must be taken into consideration on several points. First, the personality, the individuality of the patient must stand out in the picture.

Secondly, they should be categorised under subjective, objective, general, common and uncommon symptoms. In fact, the similimum is practically never found amongst the disease symptoms.

In considering the disease symptoms in the selection of remedy, its only practical value is in excluding those remedies from consideration which do not correspond to the genius of the disease, but act chiefly on other parts of the organism.

Thee are different methods of evaluation of symptoms devised and formulated by various pillars of homoeopathy.

    1. **Kentian method:** According to this, highest emphasis is given to the mental generals reflecting the innermost of the patient.

    2. **Hahnemann's method:** It categorises the symptoms into general and uncommon types out of which the uncommon ones get a higher value.

    3. **Garth Boericke's method:** It classifies the symptoms as basic or absolute and determinative types.

    4. **Boenninghausen's method:** It consists of the following.

a.   **Quis:** It includes the personality of the patient which deals with age, sex, body build, constitution and temperament

b.   **Quid:** It deals with the nature of disease.

c.   **UBI:** It means seat of disease.

d.   **Quibus auxilus:** It means the associate symptoms with the main complaint.

e.   **Cur:** It deals with the cause of disease.

f.   **Quomodi:** The modifying factors which increase o

decrease the intensity of complaints such as weather changes, time of the day, eating habits, etc.

g. **Quando:** It mainly deals with the evolution of disease.

Q-1. Give the scheme of evaluation and gradation of symptoms according to Kent. (1988,1990)

A-1. Dr. James Tyler Kent was the first to introduce the scheme of analysis, evaluation and gradation of symptoms to reach the similimum.

Evaluation: It implies the principle of ranking of different symptoms in order of value which are to be matched with the drug symptoms.

As a result of painstaking enquiry the physician has accumulated a mass of data which threatens to engulf him. He has to classify them in order to give it a form. This form will have to depict truly the patient as a person, which at the same time will readily reveal its counterpart in materia medica. This classification is accepted as the evaluation of the case.

KENTIAN FEATURES OF EVALUATION:

1. Prime importance to the mental state.
2. Limited generalisation.
3. Physical generals including modalities.
4. Characteristic particulars considered at the final stage of differentiation.

Scheme of evaluation: The symptoms have been classified as:
1. General symptoms.
2. Common symptoms.
3. Particular symptoms.

1. **General symptoms:** For details see Q-1 Chapter-3. P-24.

2. **Common symptoms:** These symptoms are common to a particular disease or are found in several patients as a common factor. They are usually of secondary importance and do not play much role in the selection of similimum, unless they have peculiar modalities.

3. **Particular symptoms:** For details see Q-5(b) Chapter-3. P-33.

Rules to be followed:

1. The generals always rule the roast.

2. The general symptom must be strong and well-marked.

3. A number of strong particulars must not be ignored on account of one or more weak generals.

4. Symptoms relating to vital organs are of more importance than those relating to less vital parts, eg:

   a. Symptoms referring to central nervous system, heart, lungs, digestive system are of greatest importance.

   b. Symptoms referring to the skeleton, muscles, joints, peripheral nerves are of lesser importance.

   c. Symptoms referring to the subcutaneous tissue or skin are of least importance.

5. Common particulars may in certain conditions assume comparative high rank

   a. by virtue of their appearance at two or more sites.

   b. as the last appearing symptoms of the case.

6. In mental diseases bodily symptoms are to be considered as concomitants, while mentals in case of physical illness for the final differentiation of the medicine.

STUDY OF REPERTORY

7. Mental symptoms aggravated or ameliorated by physical generals are of high rank.

GRADATION ACCORDING TO DR. KENT:

Gradation is the ranking of the symptoms according to their importance. The symptoms are ranked in the following grades.

1. **First grade:** The symptom that appeared in majority of provers, confirmed by several reprovings and verified upon the sick. It is printed in the Kent's Repertory in capital.

2. **Second grade:** These symptoms were brought out by few provers, were confirmed by reproving and ocasionally verified upon the sick. They are printed in the Repertory in italics.

3. **Third grade:** They are the symptoms of lowest rank. These symptoms were brought out by only few provers, not confirmed by reproving or verified by curing a patient; but they stood very prominently in the affected provers. They are shown in the Kent's Repertory in plain or Roman type.

Q-2. What is the need of evaluation of symptoms? Describe the evaluation of symptoms according to Dr. Kent. (1988 supp)

A-2. The evaluation usually deals with the ranking of the symptom. It has to be done effectively.

Need for evaluation: A case is full of symptoms of which all are not of same importance and value. Therefore in order to reach the similimum the symptoms have to be arranged accordingly.

For second part see Q-1 chapter-4. P-36.

Q-3. What is meant by gradation? Explain in how many grades the symptoms are divided? Describe each (1986)

A-3. See Q-1 Chapter-4. P-36.

Q-4. Write short notes on:

a. Modality (1987)

b. Peculiar symptoms (1986, 1990)

c. Place of mental symptoms in repertorisation (1985, 1989)

d. Totality of symptoms (1989)

e. Key-note symptoms (1989, 1990)

f. Kinds and sources of general symptoms (1986, 1989)

g. Prescribing symptoms (1990, 1992)

A-4. Modality: By modality we mean the circumstances of aggravation and amelioration of any abnormal sensation felt by the patient. Amongst the modalities causative factors, predisposing as well as the precipitating rank first, the aggravations come next while the ameliorations are taken last.

Thus from the standpoint of individualisation modalities assume the highest importance and the success of the prescription depends upon the ability of the homoeopathic physician to evaluate them correctly.

They can be of various types:

1. **Time modality:** Worse 4-8 P.M. - Lycopodium; 10-11 A.M. - Nat mur.

2. **Postural modality:** It relates with the physical position.

    a. Better in knee-elbow position - **Medorrhinum.**

STUDY OF REPERTORY

   b. Worse by standing - Sulphur.

   c. Better by absolute rest and lying on painful side - Bryonia.

3. **Circumstantial modality:** It usually deals with the circumstances, or the place.

   Anxiety with anger - Sepia.

4. **Seasonal modality:** It relates with a particular season or weather.

   a. Better in damp weather: Causticum, Nux vomica, Hepar sulph, Medorrhinum.

   b. Worse in damp weather: Nat sulph, Thuja, etc.

   c. Worse during winter: Silicea, Calc carb, etc.

   In this way modalities are helpful in guiding towards the selection of similimum.

   Peculiar symptoms: See Q-4 Chapter-3.

   Place of mental symptoms in repertorisation:

   See Q-3 Chapter-3.

   Totality of symptoms: It is not merely a haphazard, fortuitous jumble of symptoms thrown together without rhyme or reason and not merely a numerical aggregate. It means all the symptoms of the case which are capable of being logically combined into harmonious and consistent whole, having form, coherency and individuality.

   Dr. Hahnemann calls the totality as **"outwardly reflected picture of the internal essence of the disease"**

   According to Dr. Stuart Close, **"Totality means the sum of the aggregate of the symptoms.**

According to Dr. H.A. Roberts, "The totality is that concrete form which the symptoms take when they are logically related to each other and stand forth as an individually recognisable form."

Sources of totality:

1. From the patient himself.

2. From his attendants, relations.

3. From the observation of the physician and the examination done by him.

4. From his past, personal, social history and background of family and habits.

It has been mentioned in Section-5 of the 5th edition of Organon of Medicine.

Keynote symptoms: See Q-4 Chapter-3. P-31.

Kinds and sources of general symptoms

For kinds see Q-1 Chapter-3. P-24.

Sources of general symptoms

1. From the patient himself.

2. From the observation of the physician.

3. From his past, personal and family history.

4. From his attendants and relations.

5. By the examination done by the doctor.

Prescribing symptoms: The symptoms on which the prescription is based are called the prescribing symptoms. Since homoeopathic prescription results from the detailed case-taking, different bases are attributed to the prescribing symptoms:

STUDY OF REPERTORY

1. **On the basis of etiology:** It means the cause of disease, acute or chronic. It can be either immediate or a remote cause.

2. **On the basis of characteristics:** It means selecting few characteristics or peculiar symptoms on which the prescription is based. They can be either physical general or mental general.

3. **On the basis of constitution:** The concept of constitution is as old as the evolution of homoeopathy. This not only means the physique but also the mental aspect with the environmental stimuli and changes affecting the personality as a whole.

It can be either hydrogenoid, nitrogenoid or carbonitrogenoid type of constitution.

4. **On the basis of pathology:** It is becoming more common in day-to-day practice. It means to **choose a specific** depending on the name of disease. For example,

Acute upper respiratory tract infection - Belladonna.

For measles: Belladonna.

5. **On the basis of miasms:** It usually deals with the miasmatic background. It can be studied by complete case-taking and analysis. They can be antipsoric, antisycotic or antisyphilitic or the combination of any two or all the three.

6. **On the basis of nosodes and bowel nosodes:** They are the medicines prepared from the disease matter, such as Bacillinum, Tuberculinum, Parotidinum, etc.

Usually if the present complaints date back to some previous acute disease then the particular nosode should be given, e.g., complaints after measles give Morbillinum, complaints after tuberculosis give Tuberculinum.

7. **On the basis of laboratory investigations:** They are on the rise, thereby changing the value of prescription in homoeopathy. For increased blood sugar give Cephalandra, for increased blood urea give Eel serum, etc.

8. **On the basis of autotherapy and autohaemotherapy:** When there is nothing to prescribe on and the patient is suffering from some chronic disease for which no appropriate homoeopathic medicine is found, then from his body blood, urine or sputum is taken and potentised according to the principles and administered.

9. **On the basis of tautopathy:** By this the bad effects of allopathic drugs are said to be antidoted. In this the same allopathic medicine is given in the potentised form.

10. **On the basis of placebo:** It is sac lac which literally means 'to please'. It is the best method of performing the act of prescribing. It should be given when there is no time to study the new case, when the case is not clear, when the symptoms have to be analysed, or when there is no need for any medication, but to satisfy the patient.

CHAPTER-5

CHOICE OF REPERTORY

Repertory is an index of the symptoms of materia medica, record of scientific provings which is reproduced and artistically arranged in a practical form to facilitate the quick selection of the indicated medicine.

Although the field of homoeopathy is flooded with number of repertories but the ultimate choice of the repertory rests on the physician himself.

The aim of repertory is never to replace the materia medica, but to render choice of a medicine easy. Thus the study of repertory helps to understand the patient and materia medica. Repertory findings may be cross-checked with the materia medica.

The final choice of repertory depends upon the type of case whether acute or chronic, on the nature of chronic disease, either with a full blown picture or only as a one sided disease.

Q-1. What is the difference between Kent's and Boger Boenninghausen's Repertory? Which one will you choose and why? (1988, 1988 supp, 1990)

A-1. Although there are many repertories in the market but the most commonly used are the Kent's and Boger's Repertories.

Every repertory differs from the other in one way or the other. These differences are only apparent although they can be explained theoretically on the basis of the principles of the repertory.

Comparison

Kent's Repertory	Boger's Repertory
1. **Fundamental principle:** It goes from generals to particulars with highest emphasis on the mental generals.	It goes from the particulars to generals with highest emphasis on the complete symptom.
2. **Sections:** It has 37 sections in total.	It has 49 sections in all.
3. **Work done:** It is done entirely by Dr. J.T. Kent.	It is a compilatory work of Dr. B.C.M.F. Boenninghausen by Dr. C.M. Boger.
4. **Highest importance:** is given to the mental generals.	It is given to the complete symptom and the concomitants.
5. **Role of concordances:** There is no definite role in the Repertory.	There is a separate chapter regarding Concordances of the Remedies.
6. **Type of gradation:** It has gradation in three classes: Grade I, II, III Bold: 1st grade Italics: 2nd grade Simple: 3rd Grade	It has gradation in 5 scales. Bold = 5/1st grade Dark = 4/2nd grade Italics = 3/3rd grade Ordinary = 2/4th grade Ordinary with Underline = 1/5th grade
7. Gradation is used both for the remedies as well as the symptoms of the patient.	Gradation is only for the remedies.

8. **Division of Repertory:** No specific division of the repertory.	It is divided into two parts. Part I= Materia Medica Part II=Repertory proper.
9. **Method of repertorisation:** Emphasis is given on the particular symptoms for further differentiation and the finest selection of medicine.	In differentiation of the remedies, and for the final selection mental symptoms are given due importance.
10. **Number of remedies:** It has about 651 medicines in total.	It contains approximately 350-360 in total.
11. **Edition:** Although in total six editions came out but the last one is called Revised 1st edition.	It has only two editions.
12. For repertorial working evaluation and analysis is very helpful.	Totality itself helps in the repertorial working.
13. Usually no principle of generalisation is followed.	It usually lays emphasis on the principle of generalisation.

14. In each chapter the rubrics with the subrubrics have been kept under the headings of side, time, modality, extension. (STME)

No such layout is seen in Boger's Repertory.

15. **Utility:** It is generally more used in cases with full blown picture where complete representation of each category of symptoms is marked. It is less time consuming and more frequently followed.

It is used in cases with pathological generals or even in one sided diseases. It is more time consuming and less frequently referred by the physicians.

The ultimate choice of the repertory depends upon the type of the case available to the physician and the availability of the symptoms. Although the choice lies entirely with the physician, he should not be biased for any particular kind.

According to the usefulness and advantages, I am mentioning the reasons to choose a particular repertory.

Why to choose Boger's Repertory:

1. **Utility in some modified cases:** The most single benefit of using Boger's Repertory is its wide applicability in the pathological diseases, one sided diseases, etc. where there are no marked symptoms.

2. **Type of gradation:** Boger's Repertory has advocated the use of 5-scale grading, they are usually indicated as 5, 4, 3, 2, 1 respectively. Although this gradation is time consuming it gives a wide range of the medicines for the selection of a final medicine.

3. **Pathological generals:** Although the pathological generals are given in other repertories also but they are beautifully represented in the Boger's Repertory.

For example, **Suppuration:** Sensations and complaints, Uric Acid Diathesis: Aggravations.

4. **Relationship or concordances of medicines:** This is one exclusive reason for the selection of this repertory. It gives a complete layout of the relationship of the medicines given in the Repertory.

5. **Complete work of Materia Medica:** As it is very well known that the work of repertorisation does not finish with the consulting of repertory and looking for the rubrics. But it needs a complete comparison of one medicine with the other which needs the help of the Materia Medica. It has been given in the first part of the Repertory itself.

6. **Principle of generalisation:** Although some physicians do not agree with the concept of generalistion but it plays a very important role. It is helpful specially in those cases where the modality of a particular symptom is not available in the repertory.

7. **Separate introduction of modalities:** It is a good layout of the Repertory that at the end of each chapter the modalities with reference to the time, circumstances, etc. are mentioned. It cuts short the time, with ready and easy availability of the symptoms.

8. **Modified representation:** Some unique features are that the chapter of fever and menstruation are beautifully modified and expanded with special additions of the constitutions, ailments related to menopause, delivery, etc. and on the complaints of infants.

9. **No need of evaluation:** It deals only with the totality of symptoms.

10. **Less time consuming:** As it does not need any evaluation or analysis, it shortens the procedure.

Why to choose Kent's Repertory:

Many repertories have been compiled by various authors in different plans and styles. But Kent's Repertory is the only one which has been written according to the scheme of Dr. Hahnemann. That's why it is the most commonly used and universally accepted repertory.

1. **Gradation used:** It uses gradation for the medicines in the scales of 1st, 2nd or 3rd grade respectively. It is helpful as it helps in judging the intensity and severity of the symptoms.

2. **Evaluation and analysis a must:** For the process of repertorisation, the analysis, i.e., division of symptoms into various groups is done following which the symptoms are evaluated for their importance and intensity. It again helps to find out the importance and the strength of any symptom.

3. **Maximum number of medicines:** Out of all repertories based on some fixed principle it is the only Repertory which gives the maximum number of the medicines on record.

4. **Systematical arrangement of rubrics:** The rubrics have been placed systematically in an alphabetical manner with subsequent placement of rubrics in the series of side, time, modality, extension.

5. **Highest emphasis on mental symptoms:** Depending on the principle on which it is based, it gives highest emphasis to the mental symptoms which reflects the innermost self of the patient.

6. **Well defined generalities:** The chapter of generalities has been very well placed and explained.

After studying the advantages of the Repertories, it becomes an independent decision of the physician to choose a particular Repertory.

CHAPTER-6

STEPS OF REPERTORISATION

Repertorisation is not only a mechanical process of counting rubrics and totalling marks obtained by a medicine, but also includes the logical steps to reach the repertory proper and finally differentiating with the help of Materia Medica.

Repertorisation uses the logic of induction and deduction. The steps to repertorisation start from case-taking and end in finding out the similimum.

The following precautions are necessary.

1. A detailed, thorough case should be taken with a special emphasis on the individual symptoms.

2. True, persistent and positive symptoms should be taken for evaluation and analysis of the case.

3. Proper emphasis should be given to the work of comparison which is done finally to select a single medicine.

Q-1. What are the various steps of repertorisation? Describe them fully. (1988)

A-1. As already learnt, repertory usage is simply not a mechanical procedure but an intelligent and scientific way of finding the similimum. The process is not an isolated one but includes various steps which have to be followed in a methodical way.

1. **Complete taking of the case:** According to Dr. Roberts "The first object of case taking is the conclusion of diagnosis" while the second and foremost one is to select the true symptoms of the patient and to clarify them so that we can make a definite picture of the illness of the patient. The presentation of the case should include the whole picture.

Recording of the case is the foremost and most essential step which gives further planning to the procedure.

For details see Q-3 of Chapter-2.

2. **Recording and interpretation:** It is difficult to keep all the data intact without any distortion, therefore the necessity of a case recording is felt. Every case can be a piece of learning therefore it should be recorded properly.

A good case record should communicate the exact and complete picture of the patient which has been obtained by the physician. It is possible only when recording is done properly without being hindered by any subjectivity of the physician.

There are certain precautions while recording the case:

1. All the events and effects should be recorded without any interpolation or deletions.

2. Do not get influenced by the symptoms of drugs recorded in materia medica.

3. Intensity of the symptoms should be given a due consideration while recording.

4. Each symptom should be valued properly with the marks against them.

For details see Q-2, Q-6 (b) Chapter-2. P-12, 21.

3. **Defining the problem:** Once the case has been properly taken and recorded, it should be interpreted in terms of the subjective sufferings of the patient. This usually deals with the differentiation of the symptoms of the disease and those of the patient.

In the language of **"Organon of Medicine"** it simply reflects what is curable in the patient. See Section-3 of **"Organon of Medicine".**

4. **Classification and evaluation of symptoms:** As we know that the symptoms are nothing but the expression of the disease and the patient himself. It is the reflection of the diseased vital force in a definite way.

The classification of the symptoms means to divide and subdivide them according to the class or the group they belong to. They can be classified into common, uncommon, generals, particulars, peculiar, rare, queer and strange symptoms, etc.

The process of evaluation means to value a symptom according to its importance and dignity. It depends on various factors like the quality of symptom, whether it is a complete or an incomplete symptom, whether modified by any influence, whether it is a single but strange symptom, etc. There are various methods of evaluation of symptoms. Some of them are discussed in brief.

a. **Kent's method:** It is the most commonly used method. Here highest emphasis is given to the "Mental symptoms".

The scheme is

1. **Mental generals:** Will (emotion, love, hate, etc.)

Understanding: Delirium, hallucinations, delusions, etc.

Intellect: Memory, concentration, etc.

2. **Physical generals:** Temperature, positions, external stimuli, bathing, any influence of season, eating, drinking, etc.

3. **Particulars:** Strange, rare, peculiar symptoms, with particular modalities.

b. Boenninghausen's method:

1. **Quis:** Personality of the individual.
2. **Quid:** It shows the nature and peculiarity of the disease.
3. **UBI:** The seat of disease.
4. **Quibus Auxilus:** Associated or concomitant symptoms.
5. **Cur:** The cause of the disease.
6. **Quomodo:** The modifying factors of the disease.
7. **Quando:** The evolution of disease with a special reference to the time of appearance, aggravation and amelioration of symptoms.

5. **Framing the totality:** Once the symptoms have been classified and analysed, next step comes to completely frame the totality and finally select the symptoms.

According to Dr. Hahnemann, "Totality is the outwardly reflected picture of the internal essence of the disease, that is the affection of the vital force."

According to Dr. Stuart Close, **"Totality means the sum of aggregate of the symptoms."**

According to Dr. Roberts, "The totality is that concrete form which the symptoms take when they are logically related to each other and stand forth as an **individuality** recognised by anyone who is familiar with the symptomatic forms and the relationships between drugs and the disease".

According to Dr. Hale, "It is the erected and framed body of the patient."

6. Selection of repertory and repertorisation paper: Once the complete totality has been framed then comes the selection of the repertory.

The final selection of the repertory depends upon the type of the symptoms selected in the final. Kent's repertorial analysis gives the highest importance to the mental generals, physical generals and then the local or particular symptoms in the given order.

Therefore, if there are abundant mental symptoms then Kent's Repertory should be selected. If the particular symptoms are in abundance then Boger's Repertory should be selected.

If the case is completely pathological then Boericke's Repertory should be looked for. If only clinical symptoms confined to a particular system are available then special reference can be given to the Clinical Repertories or Regional Repertories.

Then comes the selection of paper. It depends on the technique of repertorisation whether thumb impression method, or complete writing of the symptoms with medicines is to be used.

7. Conversion of symptoms into rubrics: The repertorial language of the symptoms is called a rubric. The next step is the conversion of the symptoms of the patient into the language of repertory. This needs a thorough knowhow and knowledge of the repertory itself.

8. Permutation and combination of rubrics: Although repertory is a big storehouse of symptoms but at times there are some symptoms which do not have the exact expression in the repertory. Then this step becomes necessary. Two rubrics which are quite similar to each other are selected and combined to give a proper simile to the symptom.

9. **Study of repertorial result:** Once repertorisation is complete, 3 to 4 medicines come in the ambit of selection. With these medicines highest coverage of symptoms along with the highest grade is achieved. From here final medicine has to be selected.

10. **Concordances:** It usually means the relationship of medicines. It is a significant step in the procedure itself. It helps in making the second prescription when the medicine has to be changed or complemented or antidoted.

In this way the whole procedure is a systematic and methodical one which leads to the selection of the final medicine.

CHAPTER-7

KENT'S REPERTORY

It is the most commonly used and followed repertory in the field of homoeopathic practice.

Dr. James Tyler Kent started his professional career at St. Louis as a physician of eclectic school. He was a great scholar and voracious reader. When his wife fell ill in 1878 she did not respond either to eclectic or allopathic modes of treatment but was completely cured with homoeopthic medicine. This converted him to homoeopathy and he took up its study.

During his time repertories of Boenninghausen and Lippe were commonly used. He liked the form and characteristics of Lippe's Repertory but he was not satisfied with the rubrics and the number of medicines.

Noticing this, he decided to work upon and produce an exhaustive repertory. The outcome was this monumental work which was first published in 1897. It was enriched with a large number of new rubrics and medicines.

Kent's Repertory is based on the philosophy of deductive logic, i.e., from generals to particulars. It has been divided into 37 chapters with 648 drugs in the whole repertory.

He has used three varieties of typography to indicate the gradation of remedies. He did not entertain probationary remedies (fourth or fifth grade) which required demonstration by reproving and clinical verification.

To lay more emphasis on the utility of the book, in the language of Dr. Kent, **"This work completes my lifetime efforts. I have rearranged and made numerous corrections in addition to adding many remedies. This book is complete."**

Q-1. Describe the arrangement of sections and rubrics in Kent's Repertory. (1986,1990)

A-1. Dr. Kent was not satisfied with the utility of the repertories available in his time. In the repertories he found that the logic of homoeopathy was not properly followed in finding out a similimum. He criticised the faulty method of giving importance to parts and overgeneralising the symptoms.

Kent's Repertory is based on the philosophy of deductive logic, i.e. from generals to particular. The generals are dealt with in depth followed by particulars and minute particulars.

Before giving the arrangement of sections and rubrics we must understand the plan and construction of the repertory.

1. Kent's Repertory is based on the anatomical divisions of the body, with exceptions of mind and generalities which appear as separate chapters in the beginning and at the end respectively.

2. It goes from the generals to particulars.

3. The order of compilation is always from more important to less important, from above down and from the most broad general to the minutest particulars.

It has been divided into 37 sections with the following format:

Name of the chapter	Page number
1. Mind	1-95
2. Vertigo	96-106

STUDY OF REPERTORY

Name of the chapter	Page number
3. Head	107-234
4. Eyes	235-270
5. Vision	271-284
6. Ear	285-320
7. Hearing	321-323
8. Nose	324-354
Coryza	325
Epistaxis	325
Discharges	329
Smell	349
9. Face	355-396
10. Mouth	397-430
Tongue	400
Speech	419
Taste	421
11. Teeth	430-447
12. Throat	448-470
13. External Throat	471-475
Neck	
Glands	
14. Stomach	476-540
Appetite	476
Aversion	480
Desires	483

Name of the chapter	Page number
Thirst	527
Nausea	504
Eructations	490
Vomiting	531
15. Abdomen	541-605
16. Rectum	606-634
Constipation	606
Diarrhoea	609
17. Stool	635-644
Urinary Organs	646-692
18. Bladder	645-662
19. Kidneys	662-666
20. Prostate	667-668
21. Urethra	669-680
22. Urine	680-692
23. Genitalia Male	693-714
24. Genitalia Female	714-745
Abortion	714
Desires	716
Leucorrhoea	720
Menopause	724
Menses	724
Metrorrhagia	729
Tumours	745

STUDY OF REPERTORY

Name of the chapter	Page number
25. Larynx and Trachea	746-762
Croup	747
Voice	758
26. Respiration	762-778
27. Cough	778-811
28. Expectoration	812-821
29. Chest	822-883
Haemorrhage	833
Murmurs	
Heart	849
Mammae	
Milk character	837
Palpitation	873
30. Back	884-951
31. Extremities	952-1233
32. Sleep	1234-1258
Dreams	1235
Yawning	1256
33. Chill	1259-1277
34. Fever	1278-1292
35. Perspiration	1293-1302
36. Skin	1303-1340
37. Generalities	1341-1423

ARRANGEMENT OF SECTIONS AND RUBRICS

1. All the rubrics are arranged alphabetically in each chapter.

2. The rubrics are arranged from generals to particulars.

3. A rubric starts with the general symptom or a state with the list of larger group of medicines. A general rubric is followed again by subrubrics.

4. It is followed in each case by the arrangement of side, time, modality and extension. This order is usually followed in each rubric and subrubric. The arrangement has been modified at some places.

For example, in the rubric pain, following is the arrangement of the order.

Pain - General rubric	S
	T
	M
	E
Parts: Different sub-divisions	S
	T
	M
	E
Types of pain:	T
	M
	E
under each types, parts:	S
	T
	M
	E

STUDY OF REPERTORY

Although Kent's Repertory is the most commonly used repertory but there are certain drawbacks in the arrangement.

1. Certain anatomical regions have no corresponding section in the Repertory, e.g., Neck which is found under Throat, External throat and Back.

2. Salivary glands are found under Face instead of under Mouth.

3. There is no section for the circulatory, glandular or nervous system as it is not based on the systems.

4. Similar or allied rubrics often appear in two or more different places.

5. Pathological diagnosis are found frequently in generalities.

6. Objective symptoms are scattered all through the book and are often small, unclassified rubrics.

Q-2. What are the various methods of using Kent's Repertory? (1988)

A-2. Once a case is taken thoroughly, evaluated and analysed then it becomes ready for the repertorisation. As we know there are many repertories, similarly with the advancement of time and knowledge various methods have been evolved starting from the oldest of chart method to the latest computerized techniques. They are called the **working methods** or **techniques of repertorisation**.

They can be done by any of the following mentioned ways.

1. **Plain paper method:** This is the oldest method being followed at places even today. It is the most time consuming and tedious work. In this a big plain paper is taken and all the medicines are written down alphabetically in an order. Then the rubrics are related and they are jotted according to the schema of medicines appearing against a particular rubric.

The medicines have to be marked with particular signs or marks indicating the gradation of the medicine. This is done in such a manner that all the rubrics can be clearly seen and the case is analysed for similimum.

2. Thumb pit or finger impression method: As the above mentioned method was tedious so gradually the repertory was provided with the thumb impression on the beginning of each chapter. It helps in easy finding of the rubrics. It shortens the time consumed and helps in the elaborative study of the case.

In this usually no paper work is required and quick reference is given to the main or impressed symptoms which are looked into the repertory.

3. Repertory sheet or chart method: This is one of the most scientifically used methods. It contains a paper with graphic square represensation. On the left side the medicines are arranged alphabetically in a series. The medicines usually polychrest which are common are placed systematically.

In this the horizontal sections are placed to write down the rubric and the page number. In vertical columns the medicines are graded and numbered accordingly.

It can easily work out a chronic case in 35-40 minutes and an acute case in 15-20 minutes.

4. Card system: Many repertories have been given a shape of card placements. But since the Kent's Repertory is very large it has yet not been given the shape of cards.

5. Computerised technique: Computers have been introduced very fast, and their effect is being observed in the field of homoeopathy also. In this the rubrics are fed in the form of programmes and their gradation. The main advantage is its least time consumption. It gives a complete list of rubrics and the medicines graded at a glance. If in future any rubrics are to be corrected or new ones added then it can be done easily.

Q-3. Describe in brief the advantage of finding a similimum from the Kent's Repertory. (1986)

A-3. Kent's Repertory is very useful in selecting a similimum. The following are the advantages:

1. **Philosophic background:** It is based on the philosophy of inductive and deductive logic. It goes from the generals to particulars.

2. **Cross references:** They have been inserted where needed.

For details refer to Q-1(b) of chapter-5.

Q-4. Give the concept of Kent's Repertory. Describe how it differs from Boger Boenninghausen's Repertory. (1985)

A-4. Dr. Kent emphasized a detailed study of the expressions of the whole person who is sick. His explanation of the principles of homoeopathy has clearly defined the guidelines in framing the totality of disease.

He gave importance to the study of all the symptoms in order to understand the disorders which take place from the centre to the periphery, from inward to outward. Kent has classified the symptoms into general particular and common to understand the person, part and the disease.

For details see Q-1 of Chapter-7, and chapter-4. For second part see Q-1 of chapter-5. P-59, 36. P. 44.

Q-5. Describe in brief a complete layout of Kent's Repertory (1985)

A-5. Ref. Q-1 of Chapter-7. P-59.

Q-6. What are the disadvantages of Kent's Repertory? or what are the critical points regarding the usage of Kent's Repertory? (1989 supp)

A-6. After the publication of Kent's exhaustive and elaborate Repertory, other repertories were used less and less. His repertory was accepted wholeheartedly. Because it is a voluminous work some mistakes are likely to occur. They are summarised as:

1. The Repertory has many clinical rubrics which are not of any use in repertorization. For example, Pneumonia, Anaemia, etc.

2. Extremities is the largest chapter but is of least use so far as the generals are concerned.

3. There are many similar rubrics which cause confusion for the beginners specially and create difficulty.

For example, fear, timidity and frightened easily.

4. Some of the general modalities which should appear in generalities also appear in parts. For example,

wetting feet agg.- Extremities.

wet feet - Generalities.

5. Some of the nosodes are not represented well.

6. There is over-generalisation especially in section of mind and over-particularization especially in extremities.

7. Kent has given much importance to the thermal reactions, but not even a single well defined rubric is given in the whole repertory.

8. Errors of misprint of remedies, even lines are missing.

9. Dr. Kent has advocated the use of bigger general rubrics to avoid the error of omission while repertorizing but at some places general rubrics themselves do not represent the medicines which are mentioned in the subrubrics.

STUDY OF REPERTORY

For example,

General rubric - Fear

Kali Carb is not mentioned although it covers the following subrubrics.

a.	At 3.00 a.m.	-	Kali carb.
b.	of being alone	-	Kali carb.
c.	of death	-	Kali carb.
d.	while lying in bed	-	Kali carb.
e.	of being touched	-	Kali carb.

Q-7. Describe the salient features of Kent's Repertory. How does it differ from other repertories? Why is it the most commonly used repertory in practice? (1989)

A-7. For part-1 See Q-1 of Chapter-7. P-59.

For part-2 See Q-1 of Chapter-5. P-44.

For part-3 See Q-1(b) of Chapter-5. P-47.

Q-8. Where will you look for the following in Kent's Repertory? (1988 supp)

A-8

S. No.	Rubric	Section	Page number
1.	Shameless in bed	Mind	79
2.	Anxiety heart	Chest	823
3.	Constipation	Rectum	607
4.	Chilblains	Skin, Extremities	955, 1304

S. No.	Rubric	Section	Page number
5.	Pain stitching liver	Abdomen	595
6.	CA Larynx	Larynx and Trachea	746
7.	Atrophy of mammae	Chest	824
8.	Abducted, lies in sleep	Sleep	1246
9.	Metastasis	Generalities	1374
10.	Late in learning to walk	Extremities	1223
11.	Nymphomania	Mind	68
12.	Desires brandy	Stomach	484
13.	Discolouration	Skin	1305
14.	Moaning during sleep	Mind	67
15.	Stricture of oesophagus	Throat	467
16.	Tendency to fall backwards	Vertigo	99

Q-9. Give in brief the history and origin of Kent's Repertory (1991 Supp)

A-9. As mentioned in the History of Repertories, Kent's work came later. Dr. Kent used Lippe's Repertory for a number of years until it was interleaved not once but thrice. He noted his own observations and experiences not only on the margins but in between the lines also. After he took up the teaching of Materia Medica in 1883, he became more convinced of the need of a better repertory.

Dr. Kent was not satisfied with the work of Jahr, and Boenninghausen. He found them unsuitable in practice. In order to compile a complete repertory he got hold of the manuscripts of most of the repertorial work.

He talked to Lee of Philadelphia as Lippe's abridged form of repertory was with him. Lippe had desired that Dr. Kent should work jointly with Lee in producing a comprehensive repertory. At that time Kent had already compiled the sections of urinary organs, chill, fever and sweat.

Dr. Kent followed the same plan and layout as in the Lippe's Repertory. He added his clinical notes especially those which did not contradict proving. After completing this work, he started using this for his own purpose. He found difficulty in publishing it on account of high cost.

At last Dr. Kimball, Thurston and Biegler helped him to get enough subscribers to justify the publication. In this way the first edition came in the year 1897. It was used extensively by the homoeopaths.

Dr. Kent was not sure whether his work would undergo a third edition. He left behind the handwritten corrected copy for the third edition on his death in 1916. Dr. Ehrhart with the assistance of Dr. F.E. Gladwin and Dr. J.S. Pugh published the third edition in 1924, eight years after the death of Dr. Kent.

The third edition was again revised, compared and corrected from the handwritten copy of Kent. The successive fourth and fifth editions were published with the help of Dr. Gladwin, Dr. Clara Louise Kent and Dr. Pierre Schmidt.

The sixth American edition was published in 1957 while the Indian edition came out in 1961.

A revised version of Kent was published in May 1974 under certain unusual circumstances. Dr. Pierre Schmidt took the pains of going throught it, word by word and detected many mistakes in the form of omissions, grading of medicines and arrangement of rubrics in both Indian and American editions.

He corrected it with the help of the original work of Dr. Kent. Unfortunately when the book was ready for publication it was stolen. Dr. Diwan Harish Chand, an eminent homoeopath of India, succeeded in salvaging the manuscripts which were in mutilated form. This is the supposed seventh edition but it is called the revised first edition. This in brief shows the ups and downs of Kent's Repertory.

CHAPTER-8

BOGER'S CHARACTERISTIC AND REPERTORY

Dr. C.M. Boger was a leading practitioner of the United States in early decades of this century.

In his time both Boenninghausen's and Kent's Repertory were popular. He made a study of both and accepted the Boenninghausen's way of working out of a case. Finding that the practitioners had to depend on the existing faulty translations of Repertory of Antipsorics he started the work of translating it in 1900.

In the course of his translation work, he was further convinced that Boenninghausen's basic principles, plan and construction were sound and that the book was very practical.

He started his work by adding up aggravations, ameliorations and concomitants in a detailed manner at the end of every chapter. It was first published by Boericke and Tafel in 1905.

This Repertory is based on the following fundamental concepts:

1. Doctrine of Complete Symptom.
2. Doctrine of Pathological Generals.
3. Doctrine of Causation and Time.
4. Doctrine of Clinical Rubrics.

5. Evaluation of Remedies.

6. Fever Totality.

7. Doctrine of Concordances.

This repertory is yet to show its efficacy in the field of homoeopathy.

Q-1. Describe the arrangement of sections and rubrics in Boger Boenninghausen's Repertory. (1985, 1991)

Ans-1. Boenninghausen's pioneering work was in great use during the second half of the 19th century. But with the publication of Kent's Repertory in 1897 it receded to the back stage. But Boger resuscitated Boenninghausen's work by refining and enriching the fundamentals.

While working he subscribed to the principle of totality of symptoms which was originally given by Hahnemann. Before beginning with the arrangement we must know the fundamental concepts of the repertory. They are:

1. Doctrine of complete symptom.
2. Doctrine of pathological generals.
3. Doctrine of causation and time.
4. Clinical rubrics.
5. Evaluation of remedies.
6. Fever totality.

ARRANGEMENT OF THE REPERTORY

1. Most of the sections in the book are starting with the **rubrics.** The location rubrics are followed by further subdivision of parts, with each part having rubrics like side and extending to.

STUDY OF REPERTORY 83

After the location different sensations are arranged in the alphabetical order. Each sensation is a general rubric which is followed by a group of medicines.

2. The medicines are grouped under the broad division of time like daytime, morning, forenoon, etc. There is no specification of hours like in Kent's Repertory.

3. There is a subsection of Aggravation which includes the factors exciting or bringing on the complaints. This subsection is larger than the amelioration and most useful for repertorisation particularly of acute cases.

4. There is a subsection of Amelioration which has the least number of rubrics. It is used only for the individualisation of the case.

5. **Concomitants:** It is one of the major contributions of Boger. Most of the concomitants are well explained and arranged in an alphabetical order.

6. **Cross reference:** It comes next to the concomitants in importance. In our day-to-day practice we get a bundle of symptoms creating confusion, with scarcity of exact repertorial expressions. But in all these conditions we have to evaluate and come to the characteristic symptoms and adequately convert them into the rubrics. Here comes the importance of cross references which helps in clearing the confusion created by similar rubrics.

7. There are following sections with the arrangement of them as follows:

MIND

Time

Aggravation

Amelioration

Concomitants

Cross-reference

Sensorium

Agg and Amelioration

VERTIGO

Time

Aggravation

Amelioration

Concomitants

Agg - Cross reference

HEAD INTERNAL

Time

Agg

Amel

Cross reference

Agg - Cross reference

Amel - Cross reference

HEAD EXTERNAL

Time

Agg

Amelioration

Cross reference

STUDY OF REPERTORY

EYES
Cross reference
Eyebrows
Orbits
Orbits - Cross reference
Eyelids
Eyelids - Cross reference
Canthi
Time
Agg
Amel
Vision
Time
Agg
Amel

EARS
Hearing
Time
Agg
Amel

NOSE
Smell

Time
Agg
Amel
Coryza
Time
Amel
Concomitants

FACE
Lips
Lower jaw and maxillary joints
Chin
Time
Agg
Amel

TEETH
Gums
Time
Agg
Amel
Concomitants

MOUTH
Palate

STUDY OF REPERTORY

Throat
Saliva
Tongue
Time
Agg
Amel

APPETITE
Time

THIRST
Time

TASTE
Time
Agg
Amel

ERUCTATION
Time
Agg
Amel

WATERBRASH AND HEARTBURN
Time
Aggravation

HICCOUGH
Time
Agg
Amel

NAUSEA AND VOMITING
Time
Agg
Amel
Concomitants
Cross reference
Agg - Cross reference

STOMACH
Epigastrium
Stomach-Epigastrium
Agg
Amel
Concomitants
Cross reference

HYPOCHONDRIA
Time
Agg

Amel
Cross reference

ABDOMEN
Time
Agg
Amelioration
Cross reference
Agg - Cross reference
Amel - Cross reference

EXT. ABDOMEN
Agg
Cross reference

INGUINAL AND PUBIC REGION
Agg
Cross reference
Mons pubis

FLATULENCE
Time
Agg
Amelioration
Cross-reference
Agg - Cross reference

STOOL
Concomitants
Before stool
Concomitants
During stool
Concomitants
After stool
Time
Agg and Amelioration
Cross reference
Concomitants
Before stool - Cross reference
Concomitants
After stool - Cross reference
Agg and Amelioration - Cross reference

ANUS AND RECTUM
Conditions
Cross reference

PERINEUM
Conditions
Cross reference

PROSTATE GLAND

Urine

Sediment

Micturition

Before urination

At the beginning

During urination

At the close of

After urination

Conditions of urination

Cross reference

Sediment — Cross reference

Micturition - Cross reference

During urination — Cross reference

After urination — Cross reference

URINARY ORGANS

Kidneys

Urethra

Bladder

Urethra

Meatus

Conditions

Kidneys - Cross reference

Bladder - Cross reference

Urethra

GENITALIA

Male organs

Penis

Glans

Prepuce

Spermatic cord

Testes

Scrotum

FEMALE ORGANS

Time

Conditions

Male organs - Cross reference

Penis - Cross reference

Glans - Cross reference

Prepuce - Cross reference

Spermatic cord

Testes

Scrotum

Female organs

SEXUAL IMPULSE

Concomitants of coition

Concomitants after coition

Concomitants after pollutions

Concomitants after coition - Cross reference

Concomitants after pollution - Cross reference

MENSTRUATION

Concomitants before menses

Concomitants at the start of menses

Concomitants during menses

Concomitants after menses

Leucorrhoea

Concomitants to leucorrhoea

Cross reference

Leucorrhoea - Cross reference

RESPIRATION

Impeded by

Time

Agg

Amel

Concomitants

COUGH

Excited or agg by

Amel

Concomitants

Expectoration

Taste of expectoration

Colour of expectoration

Odor of expectoration

LARYNX AND TRACHEA

Agg

VOICE AND SPEECH

Time

Conditions of voice

NECK AND EXTERNAL

Throat

Nape

Time

Agg

Amel

CHEST INNER

External

STUDY OF REPERTORY 95

Axillae
Mammae
Nipples
Heart and region of mammae
Agg
Amel

BACK REGION SCAPULAR
Back proper — Dorsal region
Lumbar region
Small of back in general
Sacrum and coccyx
Spinal column and vertebrae
Time
Agg
Amel

UPPER EXTREMITIES
Time
Agg
Amel

LOWER EXTREMITIES
Time
Agg
Amel

4 F.

SENSATIONS AND COMPLAINTS IN GENERAL

GLANDS

BONES

SKIN AND EXTERIOR BODY
Agg
Time

SLEEP
Positions during
Walking
Dreams
Agg

FEVER
Pathological types
Blood
Circulation
Palpitation
Time
Heart beat
Pulse
Time
Agg

CHILL

HEAT AND FEVER IN GENERAL

SWEAT

COMPOUND FEVERS
Beginning with chill
Beginning with shivering
Beginning with heat
Beginning with sweat

CONDITIONS IN GENERAL
Time

CONDITIONS OF AGG & AMEL IN GENERAL

CONCORDANCES

Q-2. How will you repertorise a case of urticaria with the help of Boger Boenninghausen's Repertory?

Explain with 2 different cases (1987)

A-2. The technique of repertorisation is similar in any method of repertorisation. But the most important aspect is the concept of complete symptom and those of concomitants.

There is no particular emphasis on the evaluation of the symptoms but only a grand totality is considered for the repertorial process.

The principle of generalisation is followed wherever applicable. The method is discussed briefly.

Take the case properly and classify the symptoms into the groups for your convenience. Take a particular symptom and convert it into the rubric corresponding with the repertory. Then look for the symptom in the local chapter and also under the chapter of either sensations and complaints in general or conditions of agg and amel in general. The rubrics are jotted with the medicines against them specified with the grade. In this way each and every symptom has to be taken and analysed in the similar fashion.

CASE-I

1. Eruptions urticarial, burning and stinging
2. Eruptions on upper extremities
3. Burning better by heat
4. Itching worse by heat
5. Desires sweets
6. Diarrhoea worse by sugar and sweets
7. Burning of anus
8. Urine smells strong.

SYMPTOMS	SECTION	PAGE No.
1. Eruptions urticaria	Skin and exterior body	953
2. Burning	Skin and ext. body-sensation	950
	and complaints in general	885

STUDY OF REPERTORY 99

3. Stinging	Skin and exterior body	953
4. Burning > by heat	Conditions of Agg and amel in general	1148
5. Itching < by heat	Conditions of Agg and Amel in general	1150
6. Desires sweets	Appetite	477
7. Diarrhoea < by Sugar/sweets	Stool	585, 606
	Conditions of Agg and Amel in general	1122
8. Burning in anus	Anus and Rectum	610
9. Urine smells strong	Urine	621

All these are taken and repertorised and the similimum is obtained.

CASE-II

A case of urticaria with stinging dryness felt all over the body. Burning in finger tips. Afraid of pointed objects; aggravated from noise, mental exertion, cold and loss of sleep.

SYMPTOMS	SECTION	PAGE No.
1. Urticaria	Skin and Exterior body	953
2. Dryness all over	Sensation and complaints in general	894

3.	Burning finger tips	Sensation and complaints in general, not available in Extremities	885
4.	Fears pointed objects	Mind	201
5.	Aggravation from noise	Conditions of Agg and Amel in general	1134
6.	Mental exertion <	"	1117
7.	Cold <	"	1110
8.	Loss of sleep <	"	1142

In this way, even if the symptom is common or particular, with the theory of analogy the similimum can very well be concluded with Boger Boenninghausen's Repertory.

Q-3. Describe in brief the distinctive advantage of finding a similimum from the Boger Boenninghausen's Repertory. (1986, 1991)

A-3. Each repertory has its own advantages and disadvantages. The basic philosophic background and the concept of totality have already been discussed.

Boger's Repertory has some distinct features:

1. Separate rubrics for affection of infants:

There is a big rubric with many subrubrics in the chapter of **"Sensations and Complaints in General."** It is a very useful chapter in clinical practice.

2. Constitutions: Different types of constitutions are mentioned in the chapter of sensations and complaints in general.

STUDY OF REPERTORY

As in the homoeopathic practice there is a well-known place of miasms and the underlying constitution whether carbonitrogenoid, hydrogenoid or oxygenoid it can be placed at the top in the list of totality and the similimum can be selected.

3. **Chapter of Fever:** This is one of the most distinctive and unique work done by Dr. Boger as an addition to the Boenninghausen's Therapeutic Book. It has many subdivisions with concomitants attached to chill, heat and sweat separately and in details.

4. **Chapter of Menstruation:** It is well organised with concomitant and conditions before, during and after menses. It has laid special emphasis on the ailments related to pregnancy, parturition and thereafter with special reference for still births and ailments from abortions.

For other details see Q-1 (b) of Chapter-5.

Q-4. How will you find out a specific remedy for a case of Headache by Boger Boenninghausen's Repertory? Explain with 2 cases. (1986)

A-4. The chapter of Head is the most elaborate in Boger's Repertory. The basic step starts with case taking and arranging the symptoms according to the intensity.

CASE-I

A case of chronic migraine in a lady of 32 years. The headache is of bursting type, violent in nature. It is aggravated before, during and after menses. Heat of sun is intolerable. Migraine usually alternates sides and is relieved by passing stools.

S. No.	SYMPTOMS	SECTION	PAGE No.
1.	Migraine (headache)	Head Internal	266
2.	Bursting	Head Internal	258
3.	Agg before menses	Menstruation: Concomitants before	678
4.	Agg during menses	Menstruation: Concomitants during	682
5.	Agg after menses	Menstruation: Concomitants after	686
6.	Agg from heat of sun	Head Internal: Agravation	290
7.	Alternating sides	Head Internal	254
8.	Amel after passing stools	Head internal: Amelioration. Condition of Agg and Amel in general.	295 1143

CASE-II

A case of Tension Headache in a young man of 23 years. The pain is felt in the whole head. The pain extends to the nose and the eyes.

There is sensation as if the head is bandaged tightly, with a feeling of a ball kept constantly in the head. The headache is worse by taking alcoholic liquors, by coughing. Whenever he fasts or does not take regular meals he feels pain, and is better by eating.

He feels relieved completely after sleep and from applying something cold on the head.

S. No.	SYMPTOMS	SECTION	PAGE No.
1.	Bandaged tightly	Head internal	255
2.	Sensation of ball in the head	Head internal sensation and complaints in general	255 284
3.	Pain extends to eyes	Head internal	263
4.	Extends to the nose	Head internal	267
5.	Headache < by alcoholic liquors	Head: Agg Agg and Amel in general	281 1119
6.	< coughing	Head internal: Aggravation Agg and Amel in general	283 1112
7.	< from missing a meal	Head internal: Aggravation Agg and amel in general	286 1118
8.	> from cold application	Head internal: Amelioration Agg and amel in general	293 1111
9.	> after eating	Head internal - Amelioration Agg and amel in general	293 1115
10.	> after sleep	Head internal - Amelioration Agg and Amel in general	295 1142

Q-5. Give in brief few reasons for the criticism of Boger Boenninghausen's Repertory. (1983, 1989 supp. 1991)

A-5. Though it is claimed that Boger's work improved and updated **"Boenninghausen's Therapeutic Book"**, but many difficulties have been noticed while using it in practice.

The following are the difficulties which have become a source of criticism:

1. The chapter of Concordances contains only 125 remedies. Though the arrangement of the remedies and construction are borrowed from Boenninghausen the number of remedies under each heading are less and for practical purposes causes difficulty.

2. In Boger's Repertory mind section has been enlarged and developed from the practical point of view. But concomitant subsections have only few remedies which make it insufficient.

3. **Misplacement of rubrics:** Many rubrics are not given at proper place thereby creating difficulty in finding them out.

4. Though it is an elaborative repertory it does not have many medicines.

5. There is over-emphasis on the theory of analogy and generalisation.

6. Nosodes are not well represented in it.

7. There are many rubrics with single medicine which create confusion and cannot be used for repertorisation.

8. Some of the information available in Synoptic Key of Boger is missing in the repertory, eg., Dreams of snake: Lachesis is not mentioned.

9. Although concomitants have been given much importance but at certain places and in some chapters they are missing completely.

Q-6. Where will you locate the following in Boger Boenninghausen's Repertory?

1. Headache better after stool (1988, 1990)
2. Pain extends upwards
3. Sneezing
4. Urination involuntary
5. Wave-like sensation

6. Hydrocele of boys
7. Hiccough
8. Backache during menses.

A-6.

S.No.	SYMPTOMS	SECTION	PAGE No.
1.	Headache better after stool	Head Internal. Amelioration / Agg and Amel in general	295 / 1143
2.	Pain extends upwards	Sensations and complaints in general	892
3.	Sneezing	Coryza	384
4.	Urination involuntary	Micturition	627
5.	Wave-like sensation	Sensations and complaints in general	934
6.	Hydrocele of boys	Scrotum	655
7.	Hiccough	Hiccough	498
8.	Backache during menses	Menstruation: concomitants during	685

Q-7. Write short notes on Boger Boenninghausen's Characteristic and Repertory (1988, 1988 supp.)

A-7. For details see Q-1(b) Chapter-5 and details of chapter-8. P-47, 71, 72.

CHAPTER-9

CARD REPERTORIES

The development and introduction of Card Repertories have their own story.

Since time immemorial man tries to find an easy and simple way to treat the human sufferings. Similarly with the introduction of Kent's, Boger's and many other repertories, it was found to be time consuming and cumbersome.

With this started the work for an easy way of finbding out the similimum. So some physicians started preparing their own chits, diaries and different types of paper cuttings. These finally gave birth to card repertories.

This method permits a considerable saving of time and gives intense degree of flexibility in the working of a case which is difficult to achieve in other methods of repertorisation.

The working with Card Repertories requires a sound knowledge of

1. The concept of totality of symptoms.
2. The classification and evaluation of symptoms.
3. Scope and limitations of the method of repertorisation.

The first card repertory came into use in 1892 when Dr. Guernsey prepared slips for Boenninghausen's Repertory.

Card Repertory is a system of visuals which eliminates the necessity of writing out the rubrics and remedies against them. It helps in the easy study and combination of rubrics.

Method of working out a case: In this, symptoms are converted into rubrics. The rubrics are seen in the Index Book, to look for the particular card number.

The cards are taken out and arranged properly. Keeping them in a series, they are seen by the light fully. It gives the indicated similimum.

GENERAL PRINCIPLES FOR THE CONSTRUCTION:

1. Important generals are used as rubrics.
2. Cards are employed to determine the likely group of remedies that closely correspond to the general picture of the case.
3. Numerical evaluation plays a little part in this method.
4. It usually suits a chronic case which presents with a changed but vivid symptoms.

SELECTION OF RUBRICS:

1. Conversion of the symptoms in the case record into rubrics should be accurate.
2. Characteristic concomitants must always be included.
3. Top priority should be given to the cause.

   Predisposing and precipitating factors, particularly in the emotional sphere, should be given due place.
4. Generalization of a particular symptom on inadequate grounds should be avoided.

STUDY OF REPERTORY

FOLLOWING IS THE LIST OF CARD REPERTORIES:

S. No.	Name of repertory	Year of publishing
1.	William Jefferson Guernsey later improved by Dr. H.C. Allen.	1892
2.	Dr. Margret Tyler.	1912
3.	Dr. Field, based on Kent's work	1922
4.	Dr. C.M. Boger.	1928
5.	Dr. Marcos Jaminez, based on Boenninghausen's work.	1948
6.	Dr. Broussalian's Card Repertory	1948
7.	J.G. Weiss Card Repertory	1950
8.	R.H. Farley's Spindle Card Repertory	1950
9.	Dr. P. Sankaran's Card Repertory	1950
10.	Dr. Jugal Kishore's Card Repertory	1959
11.	Dr. Shashi Mohan Sharma's Card Repertory	1984

Q-1. What is the advantages of Card Repertories? Describe few card repertories you know. (1988)

A-1. Card repertories: It is a system of visual sorting and helps the physician by eliminating the necessity of writing out the rubrics and remedies.

Although there are book repertories in the market but card repertories have their own merits and demerits.

ADVANTAGES OF USING A CARD REPERTORY:

1. **Less time consuming:** In the fast, mechanical world of today other methods become very time consuming and haphazard. But with the entry of card repertories the procedure of repertorisation has become less time consuming.

2. **No need for analysis and evaluation:** There are some repertories which usually require the placement of symptoms in a graded or evaluated manner which itself is time consuming. But the use of card repertories does not require it at all.

3. **A clear, modified concept of totality:** There are many principles of using a repertory. But the operation of card repertory demands only a correct totality which can be used for the purpose of repertorisation.

4. **Simple to operate:** The procedure of using the card repertories is so simple that even a layman can use it. There is no need to convert the symptoms but only peeping into a particular card for the requirement of a particular symptom; then separating the cards, arranging them and looking for the similimum.

5. **No paper work:** The other repertories require a lot of writing and paper work which in fact is not needed by this method, which makes it to some extent economical.

6. **Limited generalisation:** This is one of the most significant uses that unlike other repertories it does not lay emphasis on the principle of the grand generalisation, which makes it more useful.

In brief we have discussed the points of utility of the card repertories. There are various card repertories. Let us consider them one by one.

1. **BOGER'S CARD REPERTORY:** It is based on the general analysis which represents itself best in the sixth edition.

In this repertory he has taken a middle ground by finding the anatomical sphere wherein the symptoms arise or occur, modifying this by modalities first and then reducing the number of remaining remedies by noting the discrete symptoms as found in Kent's repertory.

According to Boger, the preliminary choice of remedies should be limited by the rubric pertaining to locations and the pathological generals.

2. **FIELD'S CARD REPERTORY:** It is also called **magnum opus** in the field of card repertories. It contains more than 6000 cards. It is based entirely on the plan of Kent's Repertory but with few additions. The remedies are indicated on the card by code numbers, a key to which is available.

An accompanying book lists only the rubrics and not the remedies. But the repertory is very cumbersome and just adorns the shelves of few who possess this valuable document.

3. **SANKARAN'S CARD REPERTORY:** It is an additional attempt of Dr. P. Sankaran to increase the usefulness of Boger's card repertory by the addition of rubrics and remedies which have been omitted in it.

4. **SYNOPTIC CARD REPERTORY:** It was compiled by Dr. L.D. Dhawle to get over the difficulties experienced by him while working with Boger's Card repertory of which he was an acknowledged exponent. It has overcome all the shortcomings of Boger's card repertory.

5. **FARLEY'S SPINDLE REPERTORY:** It is based on the philosophy of Dr. Kent. This repertory does not get over the paucity of general rubrics and at places omits some remedies which should have got in. Nothing much is known about this work.

6. **KISHORE CARD REPERTORY:** This repertory was compiled by Dr. Jugal Kishore in 1959. It has nearly 10,000

cards in it. It is entirely based on the framework of Kent's repertory. Earlier there were 3500 cards but now the number has been raised to 10,000 with 600 medicines in it. The special feature of this repertory is the use of gradation of medicines in the form of different types of punched holes.

Q-2. What do you understand by the card repertories? Discuss about it in brief. How does it differ from other repertories? (1986, 1990)

A-2. Card repertories: It is based on the punch card system for listing and sorting of data. It is a system of visual sorting and helps a physician by eliminating the necessity of writing out the rubrics and remedies against them. In this the cards punched for remedies indicated for a rubric are placed one over the other so that the remedies common to the set of selected rubrics are seen right through.

It is of historic interest to find out who was the first to think of this type of mechanical elimination in the work of repertory.

The earliest work was done by Dr. William Jefferson Guernsey. He had already made substantial contribution to the literature of repertory. He had prepared short repertories on diphtheria, urticaria, throat, mastitis, etc.

He prepared Guernsey's Boenninghausen slips. They were long cards of 1-1/4 x 12-1/2 inches. It was a collection of 2500 cards being arranged in the alphabetical manner. The code number representing the rubric was kept on the top. There was a separate index where the coded rubrics were given on each card. The remedies had numbers 1-4 printed against them depending upon the degree of evaluation of that particular drug and for that particular symptom. The rubrics were chosen from the index and the indicated slips were taken out and made to lie side by side so that name of each remedy ran in a straight line from left to right. On adding up the exponent of several remedies, one with the highest number is the possible remedy for the case.

STUDY OF REPERTORY

In this way, the work was improved gradually with additions and modifications thus paving the way for better card repertories. For details refer to the introduction of the chapter.

Although there are many repertories in the market, yet the differences will be considered in relation to the commonly used and followed repertories like Kent's repertory and Boger Boenninghausen's characteristics and repertory.

CARD REPERTORY	BOOK REPERTORY
1. **Principle:** No fixed principle but only a modified concept of totality.	They are based on the principle of generals to particulars (Kent's). From particular to general (Boger Boenninghausen's)
2. **Gradation:** No gradation of the medicines.	They are graded as 3,2,1 in Kent's repertory and 5,4,3,2,1, in Boger's Repertory.
3. **Process of repertorisation:** It is less time consuming.	It is little cumbersome and takes more time.
4. **Analysis and evaluation:** It is not needed.	They are evaluated according to their importance.
5. Card repertories are more costly therefore not economical.	They are cheap as compared to the card repertories.
6. They are simple to operate and laymen can also handle them.	They are tedious to operate and needs a proper knowledge of the principles of repertorisation.

7. They are difficult to maintain.	They are simple and easy to maintain.
8. The number of cards representing the rubrics is more with the addition of rare remedies.	The number of rubrics and the medicines representing them are less.
9. They are not used as frequently as the other repertories.	They are used more frequently.
10. They are suited to the cases with full blown generals.	They are suited to almost all type of cases.
11. There is no role of grand generalisation.	It is particularly emphasized in Boger's repertory.
12. The layout basically gives emphasis on generals	It lays emphasis on both generals and particulars.
13. No paper work is needed.	It requires a complete paper work.

Q-3. Discuss the use of Card Repertories in brief. Give the salient features required for the proper selection of cards. (1985, 1990)

A-3. For part I kindly see Q-1 of Chapter-9. P-97.

The following are the salient features needed for the proper selection of cards.

1. Important generals are used as rubrics as the cards are punched for remedies with higher evaluation like 3 and 2 from

STUDY OF REPERTORY

Kent's repertory. It is essential because inclusion of the remedies evaluated low will make visual sorting well nigh impossible.

2. The cards are employed to determine the likely group of remedies that closely correspond to the general picture of the case.

3. Further differentiation in this group is not attempted with the cards. For further differentiation consult full list of remedies mentioned by Kent.

4. As particulars are employed for the finer differentiation in the group determined by the generals of a case it will become obvious that particular rubrics have no place in this method.

5. Since numerical evaluation plays a little role, so no advantage by indicating on the cards the evaluation of remedies.

6. Limited generalisation in which only those sensations and modalities that are experienced in more than two localities are generalised has to be adhered to strictly in view of the selective list of remedies punched on the cards.

7. A case with weak generals and strong particulars will be quite unsuitable for working with a card repertory. Therefore it suits best for the chronic case.

Q-4. Write Short notes on:

a. Requisites of a good Card repertory (1984, 1986)

b. Card Repertories (1988 supp, 1989)

c. Disadvantages of card repertory. (1982, 1984, 1989 Spp.)

A-4.

a. Requisites of a good card repertory.

1. The cards should be of a standard texture and thinness so that they go through the standard machines.

2. They should be strong as well as thin enough so that one or two blocking cards should not shut off the light completely when the approved cards are held against light.

3. The punching should follow the usual standards so that machines are able to punch or sort them automatically.

4. The card system should be elastic so that new rubrics could be introduced or new remedies added if needed.

5. The card system should be made comprehensive so that maximum demands of the repertorial analysis can be met.

6. The rubrics should be so arranged that it takes minimum time to sort them out from the index.

7. There should be a provision for cross reference.

8. The punching on the cards should be able to indicate the degree or valuation of drugs if desired in a particular rubric.

b. Refer to Q-1, 2, 3 of Chapter-9. P-97, 99, 102.

DISADVANTAGES OF CARD REPERTORY

c. Although the card repertories have their advantages but there are few disadvantages also. They are as follows:

1. No gradation: There is no role of the gradation of medicines.

2. They are difficult to maintain.

3. It lays emphasis only on generals, no particulars.

4. They are not cost effective.

5. Difficulty with the cards: It is deficient particularly in the quality of cards, quality of punching, etc.

6. Cross references are not properly mentioned in the index.

7. Not suitable for one-sided cases or the cases with particulars only.

CHAPTER-10

REPERTORY IN GENERAL

Homoeopathy is a science to experiment upon and an art to practice on the human beings. The methodology deals with the multiple type of symptoms ranging from those of mind to toe which can be significant as well as vague from the point of totality of the patient.

The literal meaning of the word **Repertory** is a storehouse, repository, as of information.

It originates from the latin word **Repertorium**. It is again derived from the Latin word **Reperire**. It means to find again.

It is simply an index of symptoms of our materia medica with their corresponding homoeopathic medicines arranged systematically.

1. NEED FOR A REPERTORY:

With the evolution of dynamic theory in homoeopathy the qualitative study of drugs and patients got accelerated. The provers recorded a mass of mental and physical symptoms.

Knowledge of such symptoms was useful for the treatment of chronic and acute diseases as well as for constitutional therapy but it became confusing for the practitioners to find out the similimum out of many similars.

Therefore a need was felt for a manual of symptoms, and the repertory was born.

2. **Limitations of repertory:** Repertory is basically an index. Naturally, it can serve only a limited purpose. It can never replace a physician's mental applications and knowledge of materia medica. If the physician does not use it judiciously it can produce blunders.

3. **Classification of repertories:** With the advent of different repertories, the confusion has also increased. About 158 repertories have been published by now. Therefore, it becomes necessary to classify them.

Although different types of classifications have been done by different authors but there is no universal method of classifying them. It will be discussed with the questions of this chapter.

4. **Techniques of repertorisation:** The method of using the repertory usually involves the techniques of repertorisation.

The techniques can be applied either by the old method or by the modern method.

The method will be explained in detail in the respective questions.

Q-1. How do you classify the repertories? Give a classification of the repertories mentioning in brief each type. (1988, 1988 Supp, 1989)

A-1. The field of homoeopathy is flooded with repertories of various types. The repertories are different from one another because of the difference in the principles and planning layout. In order to study them properly they can be classified into various groups.

1. **BASED ON THE PHILOSOPHIC CONCEPT:** This is one of the common ways by which they can be grouped. These repertories have a definite philosophical principle on which

they are based. The cases have to be selected accordingly so that they fit into the particular repertory. This group can be further subdivided into

a. **From generals to particulars:** In this, the generals assume more importance as compared to the particulars. For example, Repertory of Homoeopathic Materia Medica by Dr. J.T. Kent, Synthetic Repertory by Drs. Barthel and Klunker.

b. **From particulars to generals:** This concept gives importance to the particular symptoms as compared to the general symptoms.

Example: Therapeutic Pocket Book by Dr. Boenninghausen.

Based on complete symptoms and pathological generals: Boger's Characteristics and Repertory, Synoptic Key by Boger.

2. **NO DISTINCTIVE PHILOSOPHICAL CONCEPT:** These repertories are generally used for the purpose of reference rather than systemic repertorisation. They belong to **puritan group.** They help us to refer to symptoms without much variation in the language of provers.

Example: Knerr's Repertory, Concordance Repertory of Mateia Medica by Gentry.

3. **CLINICAL REPERTORIES:** They are now very commonly used for clinical pathological generals. These repertories have the basic layout in the form of systems of human body under which the rubrics have been placed. They are more a therapeutics than a repertory.

For example:

1. Berridge's Eyes.

2. Morgan's Urinary organs.

3. Minton's Uterus.

4. Bell's Diarrhoea.

5. Allen's Repertory of Intermittent Fever.

6. Robert's Rheumatic Medicines.

4. CARD REPERTORIES: They are the short cut methods of repertory for finding out the similimum. The slips of the cards are arranged systematically to facilitate the work of finding out the remedies.

1. Kishore Card Repertory.

2. Field's Card Repertory.

3. Boger's Card Index.

5. MECHANICALLY AIDED VISUAL REPERTORY: They are mechanical devices which neither need any writing nor any paper work. The work is all automatic. The marks are denoted by three different colours and the procedure is visual.

For example:

Dr. Patel's Autovisual Homoeopathic Repertory, computer repertory.

Q-2. What is repertorisation? Give a brief history of evolution of homoeopathic repertorisation. Enumerate few homoeopathic repertories which are used in practice. (1985)

A-2. The technique of working with the aid of a repertory to find out a similimum is called **repertorisation.** It is not a mechanical process simply of counting rubrics and totalling marks obtained by a medicine but also includes the logical way to differentiate one remedy from the other by the application of the **logic of induction and deduction.**

For details of evolution refer to Q-1 of Chapter-1. P-1.

STUDY OF REPERTORY

For 3rd part see Q-1 of chapter-10 and Q-1 of chapter-1. P-106.

Q-3. Write in brief the advantages and disadvantages of using a repertory in practice. (1985, 1989 Supp.)

A-3. Advantages of repertory:

1. **To find out the similimum:** The search of the similimum is the ultimate in the field of homoeopathy. This is simplified by the aid of repertory.

2. **To study Materia Medica:** The repertories are prepared from the materia medicas with a treasure of invaluable symptoms. It is the best source of all information at one place. Any drug can be completely studied with the help of a repertory moreover it strengthens and improves the knowledge of materia medica.

3. **As a reference book:** It is not easy for the physician to remember all the symptoms. So it can be used as a ready reckoner.

4. **To find out a complete symptom:** The symptoms are scattered here and there in the repertory in the form of rubrics and subrubrics. These symptoms can be assembled into the category of complete symptoms with the help of the repertory.

5. It suggests related remedies which can be useful for the selection of a drug for the second prescription.

6. It generally narrows the field for selection of remedies.

7. It helps to study all the symptoms in a sequential order that usually appear in a chronic case.

8. It gives an access to rare remedies and rare rubrics which can be valuable information for the physician.

9. With the availability of gradation of the medicines the intensity of the symptoms can be studied easily and in a comparative manner.

10. It helps to sort out those symptoms belonging to the disease and to consider only those which lie outside of the disease.

11. It helps in the individualisation of the patient by giving a group of remedies.

12. It teaches the physician to be careful in the selection of remedy and avoid routinism.

13. It helps in formulating questions which can strengthen the art of case-taking.

14. It helps in simplifying the work of the physician.

15. It helps in keeping our prejudice in abeyance regarding our tendency to prescribe on one or two characteristic symptoms.

16. It helps and improves the research job.

DISADVANTAGES OF USING A REPERTORY: We have considered the advantages in detail, let us consider the disadvantages in brief.

1. It gives only a group of medicines, not the similimum.

2. Different repertories by different authors are based on their own philosophy and follow their own plan of construction. Thus each repertory has its own limitations.

3. No repertory is complete by itself.

4. There are many rubrics which are not placed or represented well in the repertory.

5. It does not help in any way regarding the selection of potency, repetition, etc.

6. The nosodes are not well represented in the repertory.

7. There are many symptoms which do not have any expression in the repertory.

8. In case of chronic diseases where the full-blown generals and constitutional symptoms are absent, a repertory may be useless.

9. Organopathic remedies are not well represented in the repertory.

10. The repertory can differ in cases where the correct case taking and evaluation gives the correct remedy.

11. It will be of limited use for the beginners who have little knowledge of case-taking, evaluation and analysis of symptoms.

Q-4. What is meant by Repertory? Write in brief about different types of repertories. (1987, 1989)

A-4. Repertory: The word repertory originates from the Latin word Repertorium. The word Repertorium is derived from the Latin word Repertus which is the past participle of Reperire. The word Reperire means reproduction.

The word repertory means a storehouse, repository. Homoeopathic repertory is not merely a storehouse or an inventory, but it indicates something more than that.

Repertory is an index of symptoms of materia medica, the record of scientific provings which is reproduced and artistically arranged in a practical form, indicating the relative gradation of medicines to facilitate the quick selection of the indicated medicines.

For 2nd part refer Q-1 of chapter-10. P-106.

Q-5. Justify the statement "**It is impossible to practice homoeopathy without the aid of repertories**". (1987, 1990)

A-5. See Q-3 of Chapter-10. P-108.

Q-6. Write short notes on:

a. Limitations of Repertory (1988 Supp)

b. Clinical Repertories (1988 Supp)

c. Concordant Repertories (1988 Supp, 1989 Supp.)

d. Scope of Regional Repertories (1985)

e. Need for a Repertory (1986, 1989)

f. Cross Repertorisation (1982, 1990)

g. Synoptic Repertory (1983, 1984)

Ans-6.

a. Limitations of repertory: See Q-3 Part-II. P-110.

b. Clinical repertories: These repertories record clinical symptoms, diagnostics and the symptoms of clinical utility. They usually list regional symptoms.

During the 20 years between 1880 and 1900 came the era of these clinical repertories. A list of them is given below:

1. 1892 Repertory of Digestive System Arkell Michael
2. 1900 " of Back Wilsey
3. 1896 " " Tongue Douglas
4. 1895 " " Spasms and Convulsions Holcombe
5. 1873 " " Eyes Berridge
6. 1880 " " Modalities Worcestor
7. 1880 Repertory of Neuralgias Lutze
8. 1873 " "Desires and Aversions Guernsey
9. 1880 " "Intermitent fevers W.A. Allen

STUDY OF REPERTORY

10.	1808	"	" Sensations as if	Holcombe
11.	1884	"	" Cough and expectoration	Lee and Clarke
12.	1906	"	" Diarrhoea	Bell
13.	1906	Clinical Repertory		Clarke
14.	1906	"	" Throat	W.J. Guernsey
15.	1906	"	" Urinary Organs	A.R. Morgan
16.	1894	"	" Labour	Yingling
17.	1894	"	" Rheumatism	Pulford
18.	1894	"	" Eczema	C.F Mills Paugh
19.	1894	"	" Headaches	Knerr
20.	1906	"	" Mastitis	Guernsey

The main advantage of these repertories are:

1. They are less time consuming.

2. They help in those cases where only pathological or diagnostic symptoms are present.

3. They help in studying a particular system in great details.

c. **Corcordant repertories:** The word concordance means a state of being of the same heart and mind, a harmony a harmonious arrangement of the symptoms. This word was first used in homoeopathy by Boenninghausen in the Therapeutic Pocket Book. The word concordance was replaced by "**Relationship of remedies**" in later editions of Allen.

a. **Gentry's Concordance Repertory:** It is a large concordance repertory in 6 volumes by William D. Gentry where the second meaning is applicable.

The symptoms in this repertory are in the alphabetical order. Here the symptoms can be found easily which saves a lot of time. It has six volumes which are in detail:

Volume-I   -   Mind and Disposition, Head, Scalp, Eyes, Ears, Nose, Face.

Volume-II   -   Mouth, Throat, Stomach, Hypochondria.

Volume-III -   Abdomen, Anus, Rectum, Stool, Urine, Urinary organs, Sexual organs.

Volume-IV   -   Uterus and appendages, menstruation and discharges, pregnancy and partutition, lactation and mammary glands.

Volume-V   -   Voice, Larynx, Trachea.

Chest, Lungs, Bronchi and Cough.

Heart and Circulation

Chill and Fever.

Skin, Sleep and Dreams.

Volume-VI   -   Neck and back.

Upper extremities.

Lower extremities

Bones and limbs in general

The nerves

Generalities and key-notes.

b. **Knerr's Repertory:** It is compiled by Calvin B. Knerr from Hering's Guiding Symptoms.

The symptoms are arranged almost in the original form without much changes. There are 408 medicines. In this repertory the gradation has 4 distinction marks:

STUDY OF REPERTORY

1. Double thick wall   - Symptoms repeatedly verified. (II)
2. Single vertical wall   - Symptoms verified by cures. (I)
3. Ordinary lines   - Symptoms more frequently verified/confirmed. (II)
4. Single ordinary line   - Occasionally confirmed. (I)
5. Perpendicular dotted lines - Very rare symptoms. ( )

c. **Scope of regional repertories:** See part (b) of Q-6 Chapter-10. P-112

d. **Need of the repertory:** Repertory is the instrument of precision. We require a repertory in order to know what medicines or medicine we have for symptoms of the case, as all the symptoms cannot be remembered and memorised.

It is an index to homoeopathic materia medica which is full of information collected from toxicology, drug proving and clinical experiences. It acts as a link between the materia medica and the disease. It does a lot in understanding the patient and the materia medica.

e. **Cross repertorisation:** The term cross repertorisation is used when more than one repertory is consulted either to help the selection of similimum or to confirm the result obtained from the use of one repertory. A case can be repertorised by any repertory provided the case has wide dimensions so that totality can be arrived at from any angle. The main purpose of this is to highlight the oneness of all repertories with regard to their objective that is to find out the similimum. It also helps in confirming the well selected rubric from any of the repertories.

METHOD OF CROSS REPERTORISATION

1. **Rearranging the totality:** In this method, the totality is rearranged according to the philosophy of different repertories.

2. **Integrated approach:** In this the totality is first taken for repertorisation. Then rubrics are referred to in all repertories to note the availability of the rubrics.

3. **Using one totality:** In this case only one totality is used, and all appropriate repertories are consulted.

g. **Synthetic repertory:** The repertory is the compilation and synthesis of all possible sources of the materia medica. It was compiled by Dr. Barthel and Dr. Klunker. The data was collected from all sources and published in 1982. The repertory is divided into 3 volumes according to the hierarchy of the symptoms.

1. Volume-I - Mental Symptoms.
2. Volume-II - Physical generals (except sex and sleep)
3. Volume-III - Sleep, Dreams, Sex.

FEATURES OF SYNTHETIC REPERTORY:

1. Data is collected from all authoritative sources.
2. It contains 1598 drugs in total, which is the highest amongst all resources.
3. All the clinical rubrics have been well represented.
4. Time aggravations are well arranged and represented.

CHAPTER-I1

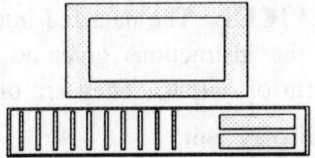

Oh! computers! you are learning computers these days. Earlier it seemed to be a strange world of speed, accuracy, and diligence. But now with the increasing pace of life, it has become a part of day-to-day life.

The introduction of computers is nothing new in the field of homoeopathy. It looks strange when the physicians take number of hours to solve a case and find out a similimum. But now with the introduction of computers it can be solved within minutes.

Let's first understand the basics of computers. The important components of a computer system can be broadly classified as —

1. **CENTRAL PROCESSING UNIT:** It is called the heart of computer system. It controls and monitors the functioning of the computer. The important parts of CPU are

    a. **Arithmetic and logical unit:** This monitors the mathematical functions and logical decisions.

    b. **Control unit:** This monitors the sequence of operations.

    c. **Memory unit:** It is the storehouse of information.

2. **INPUT DEVICES:** They are the devices to feed in the necessary information to the computer. They can be of various types.

a. Keyboard.

b. Floppy disks.

c. Tape drives.

3. **OUTPUT DEVICES:** The data fed into the computer are processed as per the instructions given to the computer and returned in the form of output. They are of various kinds.

a. Visual display unit.

b. Printers.

c. Tapes.

4. **MEMORY**: The information fed to the computer is stored in its memory. The capacity of its memory is usually expressed in kilobytes or megabytes. When a large quantity of data is handled, it may not be possible to store the entire data on the memory of computer. In such cases the data are stored on magnetic tapes, hard disks, floppy disks, etc.

5. **COMMUNICATION WITH THE COMPUTER:** The computer cannot act on its own. It only carries out the instructions given it truthfully and in the sequence given. This sequence of instructions given to the computer is called a **program.**

The computer cannot understand the language in which we communicate. The language understood by the computer is called machine language. Some languages which are commonly used are

1. Fort Ran   (Formula Translator)

2. Cobol   (Common Business oriented Language)

3. Basic (Beginner's all-purpose symbolic instruction code)

4. Pascal

6. **COMPUTER GENERATIONS:** The machinery and the peripherals of the computer system are known as hardware.

STUDY OF REPERTORY 131

The computers have been classified in the terms of generation. Let us see the four generations of computer and their components.

1. First generation - Vacuum tubes
2. Second generation - Transistors
3. Third generation - Integrated circuits
4. Fourth generation - Very large integrated circuits.

7. SOFTWARE: The series of instructions in the form of programs written and run on a computer is called the software. They are of various types:

1. SYSTEM SOFTWARE: A set of prewritten programme incorporated into the memory of a computer, by the manufacturer is called the system software.

For example:

a. operating system
b. language compilers
c. interpreters.

2. Application software: The set of programmes written for the use of the consumer is called the application software.

The introduction of computers in the field of homoeopathy is very well appreciated but the acceptance is not as quick as it should have been.

There are different computer repertories.

They are :

1. Kentopath
2. Hompath S^T
3. Medical Expert System
4. Homeonet

Let us consider a few of them in details:

1. **HOMPATH** ᔆᵀ: It was introduced by Dr. Jawahar Shah of Bombay. It has the following salient features.

    a. **Compression:** It has 7 repertories in less than 4 megabytes of space. It shows 1,500,000 symptoms and 3,50,000 references in just 3 floppies. It is thought to be the most compressed software in the world.

    b. It is the only programme which guides thoroughly to reach the similimum. It also helps in the repetition of medicine, selection of right potency.

    c. The different criteria of repertorisation can be taken depending on the type of or the mode of prescription you want to make.

    d. Thousands of symptoms can be searched easily.

    e. Graphical representation is very well represented.

    f. Comparison of remedies can be done at a glance.

    g. The prescription can be confirmed by comparing from four different materia medica.

    h. More than 125 therapeutics and differentiation of more than 125 commonly occurring diseases have been incorporated.

    1. Standard values of pulse rate, respiration rate, nutritive values, blood pressure, calorie contents, etc. have been given.

    j. 10,000 cross references have been mentioned.

2. **HOMEONET:** It is the international computer network for homoeopaths with sophisticated telecommunication facilities extending to seventy countries.

3. **MEDICAL EXPERT SYSTEM:** This expert system is written in **Fox Pro package.** It consists of nearly 85,000 lines, 400 procedures and 850 windows. Throughout the programme, the screen shows all the contents of mind, head, eyes, vision, hearing, etc. The selected option shows about 70,000 rubrics in

total. Throughout this programme, the questions and responses from the expert system are presented as screen diagrams.

The basic advantages of this system are:

1. It is a unique interactive system, i.e., you can use question-answer technique in it.
2. Repertorisation is instant.
3. Easy facility to add new rubrics.
4. Rapid repertorial analysis.
5. Storage of case records, with follow ups and their ready recall at a moment's notice.
6. Facility for searching rare symptoms.

FEW CONDITIONS OF NECESSITY FOR COMPUTER FUNCTIONING:

1. The room temp should be 15° C to 30° C.
2. Proper maintenance.
3. Use of virus guard to protect programme from fading. Viruses are able to corrupt all the data as well as the machine.
4. Avoid inserting outsider's floppy in your computer.